Be
incredibly
healthy

D1392708

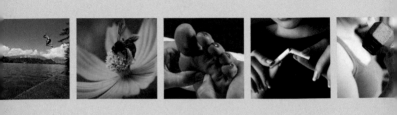

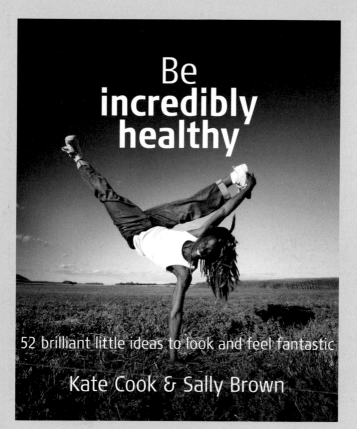

Be
incredibly
healthy

52 brilliant little ideas to look and feel fantastic

Kate Cook & Sally Brown

brilliantideas

(o13

HEA

CAREFUL NOW

If you try out even a few of the tips in this book your health and well-being should improve. However, do remember that this advice should not be considered a substitute for the help you can get from your GP. Please talk to a trained and accredited professional if you're planning on changing your diet, taking any supplements or remedies or starting a new exercise regime.

Although all website addresses were checked before going to press, the World Wide Web is constantly being updated. This means that the publisher and author cannot guarantee the contents of any websites mentioned in the text.

Infinite ideas would like to thank Clive Hopwood, Peter Cross, Dr Rob Hicks, Sally Brown, Kate Cook, Dr Ruth Chambers and Elisabeth Wilson for their contributions to this book.

First published in 2007 by
The Infinite Ideas Company Limited
36 St Giles
Oxford, OX1 3LD
United Kingdom
www.infideas.com

A CIP catalogue record for this book is available from the British Library
ISBN: 978-1-905940-23-3

Brand and product names are trademarks or registered trademarks of their respective owners.

Designed by Baseline Arts Ltd, Oxford
Typeset by Sparks, Oxford
Printed in China

Brilliant ideas

Introduction

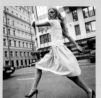

Not so long ago people often talked about healthy lifestyles, an expression that still smacks of soap-powder people in white clothes with gleaming smiles on their way to play tennis, swim or kite surf. It seemed that a healthy lifestyle was all about losing weight, building muscle, doing everything in moderation and above all smiling smugly at everyone else in order to convince them of your superiority. This is all fine if that works for you, but what it doesn't really encompass is the idea that real health is a matter of mind as much as a matter of muscle. What this book is about is total wellbeing, inside and out, and as such it includes physical fitness, diet and nutrition and also the psychological side to all of these elements. This book is about the tricks that help you to keep going, eat better and most of all beat the stresses of modern life. The ideas in here aren't just about avoiding saturated fats, they're about helping you to identify and reach your goals.

This is a book for the modern age in which the demands of friends, family and careers threaten to swamp most of us. Yet the media never seems to run out of superpeople – supermodels, supermums, superstars – all of whom only seem to exist to show us up by deftly juggling jobs, families and fitness and sporting astonishing physiques. Nobody can promise to turn you into a superbreed, but with a bit of help you can learn to stop worrying about other people's definitions of success and focus a bit more on taking the time to take care of yourself.

By learning to appreciate yourself, take care of yourself and even better yourself, you'll be far better placed to help others in their lives. Therefore a little bit of selfishness on your part can truly be the best thing for everyone else you know. You don't need a new face, body or lottery win to have a better life. Instead you can do it by simply examining your daily habits, your food, your sleep and even your bowels, and learning the little miracles that can transform every day into a better one. On the way you'll learn how to look better, feel better and stress less. You'll learn to develop a clearer idea of what really matters to you in life and what things you should simply delegate to others so they can help you achieve your own total wellbeing. Just one good idea can point you in the right direction. Fifty-two of them should help point you firmly on your way!

1. Alimentary, my dear Watson

A quick tour of how your digestion works is a useful foundation to health and a great ice-breaker at parties.

We all know that what goes in at the top comes out in a different form at the bottom. But what happens in between?

Mmmmm …

When you smell those cooking aromas, powerful chemical messages prepare you to digest your food. Chewing food gets your enzymes ready for work as the food is passed into the stomach – a soft-walled concrete mixer, churning your food in a soup of hydrochloric acid. This stomach acid is crucial: poor digestion may mean you don't have enough. Relax at meal times (stress shuts down your digestive enzymes) or get advice from a qualified nutritionist.

Gut feeling

Now on to your small intestine, which is anything but small. Your food is completely digested here, helped by

Here's an idea for you...

Give your liver a holiday by taking the herb milk thistle to help it function better, and drink beetroot juice, a liver cleanser.

Defining idea ...

the pancreas, which neutralises the acid and secretes enzymes. To help here, try food combining. Eat carbohydrates and proteins at separate meals, and fruit away from other food.

Liver little longer

It's your liver – a wonder of engineering – that gets the hardest time of all. It helps to emulsify fats and it breaks down hormones, including cholesterol. Your liver manufactures 13,000 chemicals! When we eat, the gall bladder and liver release bile which helps emulsify fats, making it easier for them to be digested. Try a supplement of lecithin, which helps your body do this.

Nearly there ...

The last bit of digestion is when what's left of your grub (mainly water, bacteria and fibre) enters the large intestine – about 12 litres (2.5 gallons) of water pass through daily. The large intestine is where friendly bacteria live. Look after them by eating vegetables and fibre, and by taking a good acidophilus supplement.

And we all know what happens next ...

2. Get smart about your heart

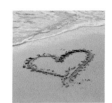

Keeping your body's powerhouse strong and healthy is easier than you think.

Heart disease is the number one cause of premature death in both men and women in both the States and the UK. But the truly shocking fact is that it's entirely preventable in all but a tiny minority of cases, with some simple lifestyle changes.

Heart disease, or coronary heart disease (CHD), to use the medical term, happens when the arteries leading to the heart muscle get furred up and narrowed. If a blood clot forms in one of these narrowed arteries, it can stop the blood supply completely, which leads to a heart attack.

So how can you stop it? As you know, cholesterol is crucial, and you need to keep an eye on your blood pressure. But the very first thing you need to do, if you haven't already, is give up

Here's an idea for you ...

Moderate consumption (one or two units a day) of red wine is thought to protect your heart (it contains phenolic antioxidants which relax the arteries). Cheers!

13

Defining idea ...

smoking. Men smoking more than twenty a day increase the risk of dying from a heart attack threefold; women smokers on the oral contraceptive pill increase their risk by ten times.

Exercise is also essential. Just twenty minutes of brisk walking, three times a week, can reduce the risk of CHD by up to 50%. Cutting down on saturated fat and eating more oily fish, olive oil and loads of fruit and veg will lower cholesterol levels and stave off the antioxidant damage that can affect the arteries. And cutting back on salt is important as a diet high in sodium (salt) is thought to be the prime cause of high blood pressure, a major contributory factor in heart disease.

But the most recent risk factor for heart disease to be identified is an amino acid called homocysteine. Taking a B-complex supplement can help reduce levels of homocysteine – and it really helps to boost your energy levels, too.

3. Dump the Marlboro man

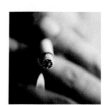

If you're a smoker, you won't need another lecture. Instead, here's some positive encouragement.

You know very well that smoking causes cancer and heart disease. In fact, most smokers actually overestimate the health risks, according to one study.

The saddest thing about this highly addictive and dangerous habit is that many smokers don't enjoy it most of the time. OK, that first cigarette in the morning, or after a meal, can taste pretty good, but after that it's never quite the same. So you light another, hoping that the next one will be better. Then the next one.

Smokers are essentially nice people with a nasty habit. So here is some good news for a change.

Here's an idea for you ...

Write a list of positive benefits of not smoking (for example, I'll find exercise much easier, I won't have to spend hours standing outside the office) and read it whenever you feel your motivation wane.

Defining idea ...

■ Have you tried to quit before and failed? Congratulations! You're one step closer to giving up for good. The average smoker quits ten times before finally managing it long term.

■ People manage to quit all the time. A lot of people are non-smokers. You could be one of them.

■ You've got a lot to look forward to. Within weeks of giving up, you'll have an improved sense of smell and taste.

■ Studies have shown that smokers on average eat less fruit and vegetables than non-smokers. Maybe eating a healthy diet when you're a smoker seems like rearranging the deckchairs on the Titanic, but you should aim for up to ten portions of fresh fruit and vegetables a day to get your maximum antioxidant protection.

■ There are hundreds of people out there willing to help you give up. Ask your pharmacist or doctor about patches and classes. Or try hypnotherapy or acupuncture.

4. What's in what?

Which foods should you target for good health? Here's a quick guide to what's in your food.

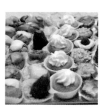

The key to a great diet is variety. This will ensure that you get a broad spectrum of nutrients – vitamins and minerals – for everyday health.

A nutritional rainbow
The rule of thumb is to eat as many different coloured foods as possible throughout the day. Coloured food is full of nutrients – look for reds, greens, yellows, oranges and all the colours in between. These will give you antioxidant vitamins that can protect you from disease.

We won't go through every vitamin and mineral here, but the B group of vitamins – found in grains and very important to our nervous system – and vitamin C – found in berries, citrus fruits, tomatoes and potatoes – deserve a special mention. Of the minerals, a key one to top up on is calcium, which is found in almonds,

Here's an idea for you …

Why not try a rotation diet? Choose a different grain for each of the five working days. So, Monday might be your wheat day, Tuesday your oat day, and so on.

Defining idea ...

'Nurture your mind with great thoughts.'
BENJAMIN DISRAELI

sesame seeds and vegetables. We need calcium for bone and teeth formation, as well as nerve and muscle function. Zinc is essential to most bodily functions, including fertility and brain function. Find it in shellfish, lentils, pumpkin seeds and eggs. And a mention for selenium which may help prevent cancer. It's naturally found in wheat germ, tomatoes, onions, broccoli, garlic, eggs, liver and seafood.

Vitamins for life
They work with enzymes to assist the body's biochemical mechanisms and helping metabolism. There are two main categories: water-soluble, which must be taken daily, and oil-based vitamins, which can be stored. The major minerals, such as calcium, magnesium and potassium, are needed either in high milligrams or even gram quantities on a daily basis. Then there are the trace elements, which are important for biochemical reactions in the body. Become deficient in any of these and eventually some part of your body will begin to grind to a halt.

5. Stress? Out!

Right here, right now, is there anything you can do to elevate your mood? Take a balanced approach.

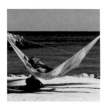

Well, one thing you can do immediately is balance your blood sugar levels. Very simplistically, sweet things or fast energy-releasing foods will send your blood sugar levels rocketing then crashing rapidly down once the hormone insulin rushes. The trick is to choose foods that sustain you. Dense, fibrous foods such as lentils do this rather than sweet or starchy foods like gluey white loaves of bread or potatoes. If not, you'll get irritable, grouchy and fatigued.

Are you intolerant?
Food intolerances, sometimes wrongly referred to as food allergies, are all the rage these days. A food intolerance can have dramatic effects – you fall down gasping when you eat nuts – or just give you a general unwell feeling or aching joints. It may also affect your mood. If you suspect you might have a problem then visit a nutritionist.

Here's an idea for you ...

Eat several snacks during the day rather than three great big meals to help you step off that blood sugar rollercoaster.

Defining idea ...

'You are what you eat.'
ANON

Fat head

Omega-3 and omega-6 fats are called essential fats because they are. Essential that is. Your body's hormones and your brain run on them so you should make sure you're getting enough. Sources of omega-3 fats include flax and hemp seeds, whereas omega-6 fats come from oily fish like sardines, mackerel or salmon.

Food and mood

Start by reducing the amount of tea and coffee you drink. Then discover tryptophan. No, it's not a village in Wales. Tryptophan is an amino acid (protein building block) that can help raise levels of the mood-boosting neurotransmitter serotonin. Foods high in tryptophan include figs, milk, tuna, chicken, sunflower seeds and yoghurt, but make sure you have plenty of B vitamins in place to process it (especially B3, B6, folic acid and biotin), plus vitamin C and zinc.

6. Walk this way

There is a good reason to put one foot in front of the other more often.

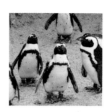

Walking is a great way to lose weight and stay slim. It is not expensive or complicated and you can do it anywhere. But there's a catch: to improve your fitness, you'll need to walk at least three times a week for half an hour a time. Here are a few other pointers to help you get going.

- You don't really need specialist gear for walking, but a decent pair of trainers will support you better than ordinary shoes.
- You'll work harder outdoors than inside on a treadmill as you'll have to cope with changing terrain and wind resistance. This is a good thing as you'll burn calories faster and get extra toning benefits.
- Wear something comfortable! It might sound obvious, but if you get wet or too hot, you'll want to give up and go back home.

Here's an idea for you ...

Don't give up on low-fat dairy products. In research, obese volunteers lost 11% of their body weight over six months on a diet that included three low-fat dairy portions a day.

Defining idea ...

'A sedentary life is the real sin against the Holy Spirit. Only those thoughts that come by walking have any value.'
FRIEDRICH NIETZSCHE

■ When walking, keep your tummy muscles pulled in to work your abdominal muscles and protect your back. Walk tall, avoid slumping and use your natural stride.

■ If you swing your arms while you walk, you'll increase your heart rate and get more of a workout.

■ For the best technique, hit the ground with your heel first, roll through your foot and then push off with your toes.

To reap the greatest benefits, set yourself a plan, say over six weeks, gradually increasing the length of time you walk and its frequency and the speed. Build up until you are walking for 45 minutes to an hour several times a week, and mostly at the faster pace. You'll be seeing a slimmer you in the mirror.

7. DIY day

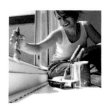

With a mass of conflicting information around regarding food and diet, there's one sure way to create a sensible eating programme.

When producing a food product, most manufacturers are trying to add value to a plain ingredient (for example, flour) by making it into something that has a high perceived value. Manufacturers also need to add ingredients that will preserve the food and stop it being a danger to the public.

This is how ingredients like trans-fats or hydrogen-hardened fat manage to creep into our food chain.

So why not step out of the food minefield by buying and cooking the ingredients yourself!

You may think that you can't possibly afford to find the time, but perhaps you can't afford not to. Start invest-

Here's an idea for you ...

For a week, try to have a different breakfast every day. You could include different types of grains such as millet and quinoa – or even mackerel on toast!

ing in your health immediately with this easy-to-do day, which will balance your blood sugar, stop cravings and take less time to do than opening a ready meal.

Have breakfast – something like porridge oats (the thick, chunky-looking fellows, not the hamster-bedding type). Shove two handfuls in a bowl then add organic milk, rice milk or nut milk (like almond or hazelnut). Here's the trick – you don't have to actually cook it: just soak the oats in the milk for a few minutes then add some chopped fruit and nuts.

Lunch could be a big, juicy salad, soup or a baked potato with cottage cheese. This is often the most difficult meal to achieve because you'll try to source it from around work. If you get stuck, cook more the night before and bring the remainder in the next day.

Dinner is easy as you largely control this yourself. It could be an organic salmon steak with steamed vegetables and sweet potatoes, or a stir-fry, or a lentil or chickpea recipe – the choices are endless. It really doesn't take long to stick a piece of chicken under the grill and steam some vegetables, does it?

8. Porridge power

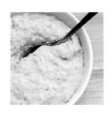

Porridge is about to become the trendiest consumable since coffee shops reinvented coffee.

In the States customers are already queuing up at a chain of cafes called Cereality to buy takeaway cartons of the stuff. Why? Here are just a few reasons.

It fights off the English
A daily bowl of porridge sustained the ancient Scots through hours of marauding. They knew that if you started the day with porridge, you didn't feel hungry for hours.

It fights off cancer
Porridge oats are packed with a rich source of cancer-fighting phyto-oestrogens, and contain an antioxidant called ferulic acid which seems to actually stop certain cancer-promoting compounds in their tracks.

Here's an idea for you ...

Bring one pint of water/milk/both to the boil. Stir in two and a half rounded tablespoons of oats. Reduce the heat, cover and simmer for fifteen minutes, stirring frequently. Add a pinch of salt.
Not hard, was it?

25

Defining idea ...

It feeds your flora

The humble oat boosts your gut flora too (you know, the bugs in your digestive tract that keep food moving through the system). Oats are a good source of probiotics, food for your body's good bacteria. The more food these bacteria have, the more they multiply – and strengthen your immune system.

It helps your heart, your blood, your cholesterol ...

Chemicals in porridge called avenanthramides stop blood cells sticking to artery walls, preventing the fatty deposits that cause heart disease. A daily serving of oats can also improve your blood pressure control, reduce your cholesterol levels and may even cut the risk of developing diabetes, by absorbing sugar from the gut and cutting the need for large quantities of insulin to be released.

... and it won't make you fat

Porridge only masquerades as stodgy comfort food – in truth, it's the nearest thing we've got to a magic diet pill. People who eat whole-grain-based breakfasts every day are a third less likely to be obese compared to those who skip the meal.

9. Geeing up for the gym

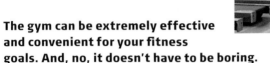

The gym can be extremely effective and convenient for your fitness goals. And, no, it doesn't have to be boring.

Have you been down to the gym recently? If not, you may be in for a nice surprise. Most modern fitness centres offer a cornucopia of classes. Go take a look …

Which gym?
Find a gym that you'll actually go to in order to keep excuses like it not being on your way to/from work at bay. Your motto should be: Location, Location, Location!

What to do?
Most gyms will provide an induction and possibly a session with a trainer – make use of this. Decide on your goal and why you're there. Is it for weight loss, for weight gain, to train for an event, to improve fitness or to build strength? Whatever your

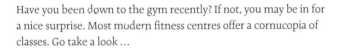

Here's an idea for you …

Get the right kit. Supportive shoes, a comfortable outfit and, for women, the right bra are a must.

27

Defining idea ...

'The worst moment in life is the moment you lose faith in your dreams. Never let it happen.'
MICHAEL COLGAN

reason, inform your trainer so they can design a programme specifically aimed at you and your needs.

Include weight-training

Weight training doesn't mean you'll end up looking like Arnie. It's a great way to add tone and definition to your body and will increase lean muscle mass, helping you to manage your weight. Using weights has the added bonus of strengthening your bones.

Have a go

Try circuit training for camaraderie, Pilates for inner strength (without having to jump around), yoga for serenity, kick-boxing to get rid of that tension, or dance to boost your sex appeal.

Three little words of advice

■ *Focus.* Get a trainer to show you your ideal training zone, or use a heart rate monitor.
■ *Drink.* A lack of water can affect your strength, stamina and ability to burn fat.
■ *Rest.* As you become fitter you may be able to train longer and harder, but muscles need rest to repair, recover and strengthen. Overtraining can deplete the immune system as well as your mood and energy levels.

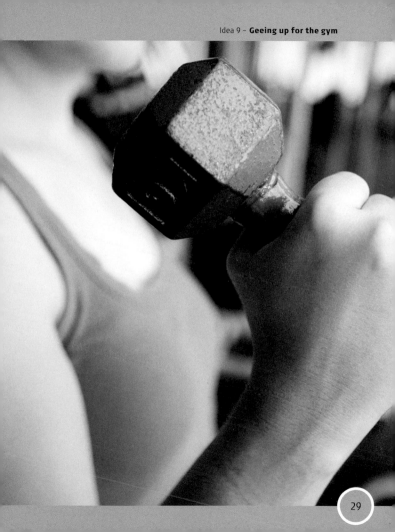

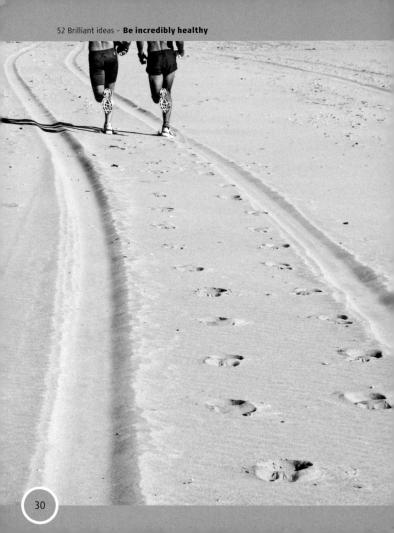

10. Get out more

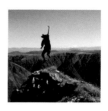

If you hate the gym, there are plenty of alternatives in the great outdoors.

Some people hate everything about the gym.
They hate the smell of them, the machines, the other people ... and no-one talks to each other because they're so busy doing exercise. And there's nothing worse than signing up for a year then never going. So instead of heading to your local exercise temple, get out and about.

Out and out good for you
Go and exercise outside. You don't have to be in the midst of the glorious countryside for this one. Your local park will do. Use the park benches to stretch, use steps to run up and use lampposts as distance markers. Let your imagination run wild.

Set goals – a good one might be to count the number of times you run round the park, each time trying to improve upon the last. Pick a route where you can see loads of wildlife,

Here's an idea for you ...

Check out psychocalisthenics (www. pcals.com). This is a form of exercise that revitalises your whole system yet takes just 15 minutes to do.

Defining idea ...

'I am at two with nature.'
WOODY ALLEN

cranes, fish, swans and ducks, even if you are in the city. What a pleasure.

The more aerobic your exercise, the better. Aerobic exercise is thought to protect you against all sorts of nasty diseases, including some types of cancers and heart disease, plus it makes your bones stronger. So do some cardiovascular stuff.

- Run, jog or walk – for at least 20 minutes each day.
- Power walking – stride out when you walk. Get into it by loading your iPod up with some seriously good music.
- Jump higher – skipping is a wonderful way to get your ticker really going. Apparently, jumping rope has the calorie-burning capacity of jogging for one mile. But you have to really go for it – no weedy jumping allowed.
- Warm up and wind down – don't forget to stretch at the beginning and end of your workouts. Warm, stretched muscles are muscles that are less likely to be injured.

11. Three's company

The best things come in threes – and the worst. Here's a basic guide to carbs, protein and fats.

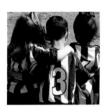

Curb the carbs?

The body uses carbohydrates (carbs) as its main fuel. Carbs can be divided into two types: 'fast burning' (junk food, processed food, honey, sweet foods) and 'slow burning' (whole grains, fresh fruit and veg, grains). The type of carbs you should curb is the fast-burning carbs because these will give you a surge of energy followed by a nasty crash. And avoid rocket-fuel carbohydrates such as white bread, white rice, cakes, biscuits and sugar. Slow-burning complex carbohydrates, however, should make up about 70% of your diet.

Perfect protein

Protein contains the building blocks (amino acids) that are used for making enzymes, hormones, antibodies and neurotransmitters as well as for repair of the body and for growth. Protein isn't just about huge slabs of juicy steak. Vegetarian sources of protein are important to consider and include beans, tofu, quinoa (a

Here's an idea for you ...

Up the amount of vegetarian protein in your diet – try tofu, lentils and grains such as quinoa.

33

Defining idea …

type of grain) and lentils. You should be aiming to get about 15% of your calories through protein, so aim to eat plenty of vegetarian sources, which are less acid forming, and also consider some cheese and eggs, but not in excess. If you eat meat, have it no more than three times a week.

Fear of fat

It's only the wrong kind of fat we should be scared of, not good fats. Saturated fats are not essential for the body to function. With unsaturated fats, there are two types: monounsaturated (olive oil is in this group) and polyunsaturated. Some polyunsaturated fats – EFAs – are good for your brain and generally make the body work efficiently. You should aim to get about 15% of your calories through good-quality EFAs. Each day, supplement with a pure fish oil and eat plenty of nuts and seeds.

12. Dare to be different

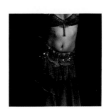

The only exercise that works is the sort you keep coming back for ... and keeping the fun factor high has real appeal.

Some people are oddly immune to the charms of the exercise bike and treadmill. They crave something more challenging and exciting. If you fancy going a bit off-road, here are some options to keep you smiling.

Belly dancing

All the sensual mystique of the East served up in gyms from Peckham to Pontefract. As an exercise belly dancing is a relatively gentle, low-impact aerobic session with a great deal of emphasis on hip movements which help tone midsections and in particular the obliques.

Pole dancing

Just in case you didn't know, pole dancing is erotic dancing using a vertical pole that runs from floor to ceiling.

Here's an idea for you ...

If you prefer the dancing part to the exercise part, try a salsa class. Smooth, sexy and relatively simple, salsa will make you fit without you even noticing.

It's a great workout too. Grabbing the pole and swinging round gives you arm and oblique strength, while more advanced moves work wonders for core strength. And the atmosphere is a riot.

Trapeze

Trapeze involves a tough upper-body workout but also a great deal of flexibility and stabilising work. The experts at Circus Space in London swear that it leads to great posture. Mainly though it's a buzz for anyone who's ever dreamt of flying through the air with the greatest of ease.

Slavercise

Following the boot camp phenomenon, a US dominatrix has marketed an alternative way to raise your blood pressure as you perform. Get ready to workout, worm. Not as yet a regular in UK gyms.

Kangoo jumping

If you ever wanted to feel like a superhero, then kangoo jumping is for you. Kangoo boots feature a spring on the sole which gives a bounce to the step. The class is a warm-up followed by aerobic moves with added boing. Currently the preserve of the more self-consciously groovy gyms.

13. Which do you want first?

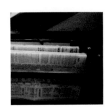

Looking for a little weight loss? Well, there's some good news and some bad news.

The bad news
If you want to lose weight, you'll need to change – and change is often hard work. That old-fashioned word 'discipline' freaks people out, but it simply means sticking to a healthy eating plan most of the time, and only occasionally going mad.

The good news
Part of the equation of weight gain is calories in versus calories expended – but only part. Gut health, the level of yeast in your system, how your immune system is functioning and your hormonal health can all have an effect on how you process the food you're eating. If you think something's

Here's an idea for you ...

Start as you mean to go on and bin unhealthy packages lurking in your cupboards and fridge. Then get hold of the right ingredients: fresh foods and basic dry ingredients like lentils, chickpeas and brown rice.

Defining idea ...

'Physical fitness isn't only one of the most important keys to a healthy body; it is the basis of dynamic and creative intellectual activity.'
JOHN F. KENNEDY

up, see your doctor or a qualified nutritionist.

The better news
There's one simple thing you need to do. Eat foods that burn slowly. This will give you sustained energy throughout the day. Ones that burn quickly rapidly increase your blood sugar levels causing insulin to be pumped into the system. The resulting drop in blood sugar will make you feel drowsy, then hungry. Insulin also stores fat, so you may put on weight if your blood sugar is rising and falling like a yo-yo.

Eat foods with plenty of fibre in them (such as vegetables), unprocessed grains (brown things), lean protein, essential fats (the clue's in the title) and slow-burning complex carbohydrates. Cut out stimulants such as tea and coffee and don't eat foods with highly processed ingredients, which means pretty much anything that comes in a box.

Nearly forgot
Exercise too. It helps the metabolic functions – breathing, digestion and circulation – to work better.

14. Under pressure

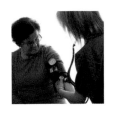

Not having a head for numbers is no excuse for ignoring your blood pressure.

Do you know what your blood pressure reading is? If not, get it checked – and write it down – then read this.

What do the numbers mean?
Your blood pressure reading is given as a fraction. In the health lottery, your luckiest number is 115 over 76; above 140 over 90, and you're in the danger zone. Blood pressure is the amount of force exerted by blood on the artery walls. The top number of the fraction refers to the 'systolic' blood pressure - the pressure exerted when the heart beats; the bottom number, the 'diastolic' blood pressure, the pressure between beats. As you age, systolic blood pressure tends to increase. If left untreated, it can actually 'burst' an artery, and then you're in big trouble.

What if your blood pressure is too high?
Drugs are effective, but you have to take them for the rest of your life

Here's an idea for you ...

Research treating high blood pressure with acupuncture indicates that it works and has a lasting effect. So as long as you're not scared of needles, give it a go.

39

Defining idea ...

and they may have side effects such as fatigue, depression and dizziness. Fortunately, lifestyle changes may do enough to help.

Eating a healthy balanced diet with at least five portions of fruit and vegetables a day and cutting back on salt is vital. Worryingly, 78% of us still add salt to our food – but even if you don't, 'hidden' levels in processed food could up your intake to dangerous levels. (Salt is called 'sodium' on the label. You have to multiply the amount of sodium by 2.5 to get the amount of salt in the product.) Losing weight if you need to, exercising more and sticking to the recommended weekly limits for alcohol will also help to take the pressure off. To really win at the numbers game, learn a relaxation technique such as yoga or meditation.

15. Space invaders

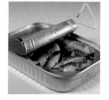

Find the space for your mind and meditate on a daily basis.

We're subject to hundreds of stimuli every day and our reactions can constitute stress. Calming the mind down is a powerful way to regain control of uncontrollable events that you could feel anxious about.

If you've ever actually tried to empty your mind for a moment, you'll have realised that it's virtually impossible. Meditation isn't about emptying the mind; it's about observation of the thoughts that are there, like watching clouds drift across a deep blue sky. The difference is you choose not to be pulled down by the thoughts by not giving them any emotional charge. It really is liberating once the penny drops that you are not your thoughts.

There are hundreds of ways to meditate. The simplest is Breath Meditation, which involves sitting quietly observing the breath entering and leaving the body. Then there's Walking Meditation, which is simply

Here's an idea for you ...

The easiest way to get into meditation is to forget books and get a CD. Amazon.co.uk have a good selection, or try your local Buddhist centre.

41

Defining idea ...

Defining idea ...

'Life is what happens to you while
you're busy making other plans.'
JOHN LENNON

observing yourself walking, mindful
only of what you're physically doing.
There is even a type of meditation
where you concentrate fully on doing
the household chores, totally engaged
in what you're doing.

Body Scan Meditation is a great one to start with. Find a comfortable
space and lie down, allowing your eyes to gently close. Be aware of
your breathing. When you're ready, bring your attention to the toes
on your left foot. Feel like you're breathing into your foot (sounds
weird I know). Work your way up your legs, through your body and
into your head. Don't leave anything out, including the naughty
bits! Spend two minutes at the end just lying in silence, then bring
yourself back to the room. The whole thing should last about 20
minutes or so and practising once a day should really make a difference. You should definitely start seeing the world through those
rose-coloured specs.

16. Take a dip

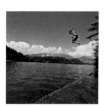

Exercising in water is like a good relationship – it's completely supportive but it also works you hard enough so that you grow stronger.

Swimming is in a league, targeting every muscle in your body while putting virtually no pressure on your joints. So if it's so great, why don't more of us do it? Basically, because we're not much good at it. Throw the average adult in a swimming pool and they do a contorted breast stroke with their head half out of the water and neck in a spasm, or a frantic front crawl that involves a lot of thrashing, kicking and head turning (and inconvenience for other swimmers).

The answer? A swimming coach will iron out the kinks and bad habits in your stroke until you're gliding effortlessly through the water. The newest teaching techniques draw on the body-alignment principles of the Alexander Technique, and the emphasis is on helping you reach a state of deep relaxation in the water.

Here's an idea for you ...

Want to instantly improve your swimming? Buy some goggles. But don't buy cheap ones –they'll leave marks on your face and fog up easily so you won't wear them.

Defining idea ...

'For each hour you exercise, you get roughly two extra hours of life.'
DR RALPH PAFFENBARGER, epidemiologist

And, because your muscles are in perfect alignment, after thirty minutes of effortless powering through the pool, you will feel like you've had a massage.

Taking lessons is also the best way to get yourself out of a one-stroke rut. Most people find one stroke suits them best and it can be tempting just to plough up and down doing it, even if it does give you a stiff neck or tired shoulders. But alternating your strokes means you will work harder, burn off more calories and target more muscles. A coach can also design workout programmes specifically for you, using different speeds and strokes as well as equipment like floats, to get maximum results. What are you waiting for? Dive in!

17. Get your nutritional act together

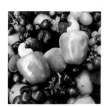

You've made the brilliant decision to take your health and nutrition into your own hands. Now what?

Put some solid systems in place to ensure that your good intentions actually get done.

Should you?
There's nothing more stressful than hundreds of 'I shoulds' running loose in your brain, like 'I really should buy fresh stuff instead of ready meals.' Write all these Shoulds down somewhere, then break them into sections, such as Diet Shoulds, Exercise Shoulds and Stress-busting Shoulds. Give each Should a priority rating from one to three and tackle the high scorers first. Only aim to take on three Shoulds a month – too many and you won't do them.

I don't like Mondays
Choose a day to start the healthy new you, but don't make it a Monday as it's always too depressing to start something when the weekend's so far away.

Here's an idea for you ..

Throw out everything in your kitchen with unrecognisable ingredients on the back of the pack – any more than three syllables and it's out.

Defining idea ...

'Be prepared.'
SCOUTING MOTTO

Take just one month at a time and say you'll stick to it for that month. If you think that something is forever, you are less likely to stick to it.

Get them in
It's time to go shopping. You'll need some of the following essentials to get you going:

- Organic porridge oats and millet
- Rice milk (an alternative to cow's milk)
- Brown rice, quinoa (a wacky kind of grain) and wheat-free pasta
- Almonds, brazil nuts and cashew nuts
- Pumpkin seeds and sunflower seeds
- Oatcakes and rice cakes
- Tahini and houmous
- Extra virgin olive oil
- Tuna in olive oil
- Lentils and chickpeas
- Tinned tomatoes, sweetcorn, butterbeans and artichoke hearts
- Dried herbs, pepper, tamari (a kind of wheat-free soya sauce), olives, pesto.

These are only suggestions, of course. You'll probably want to add other stuff and take away anything you don't like. And load the fridge with plenty of fresh vegetables, the freezer with frozen ones (better than none).

18. Ready for a detox?

Detox is such a big buzz word these days, but what exactly does it mean?

Doing a detox diet isn't quite as simple as you might think. If you're drinking lots of alcohol, simply eliminating the booze for a few days might constitute a detox diet. To someone who already has quite a pure diet, however, eliminating wheat and dairy might be a detox. Taking stock of where you are is important because if you detox too quickly you could experience a number of unpleasant symptoms, such as headaches, lack of energy and generally feeling unwell.

Don't make me

Why should we put ourselves through a detox? Our bodies are in a constant state of renewal at cell level, but if there's an overload of toxins either from food or environmental sources our bodies struggle to deal with them. That puts a strain on the kidneys and

Here's an idea for you ...

Get a juicer and start making your own juice. Juices can be full of vitamins and minerals that help the detoxification systems important to the body.

47

Defining idea ...

'The world is round and the place which may seem like the end may also be the beginning.'
IVY BAKER PRIEST

liver and takes away energy that could otherwise be used for living. A detox diet allows us to stop overloading the body with harmful substances and, if we give the body plenty of the right nutrients, it can speed up the elimination of toxins and promote cell renewal.

Be a slow starter
If you're afraid of becoming Mr or Mrs Fuzzy Potatohead, then start slowly over a period of one month. Choose in the first week to eliminate coffee, chocolate and cola, replacing them with lots of water and herbal teas. In the second week, try substitute wheat products (cakes, biscuits, pasta) with rye bread or other grains such as brown rice, quinoa, buckwheat or millet. In the third week, try substituting bovine dairy products with sheep and goat products. And in the fourth week, increase your water intake up to at least 2 litres (3.5 pints) a day, while avoiding alcohol.

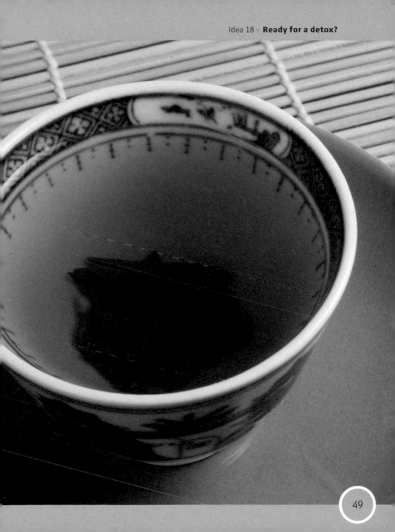

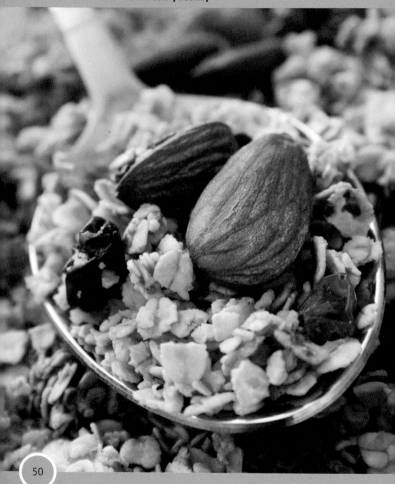

19. The incredible bulk

So what, you may well ask, is the point of fibre? How long have you got?

Generally people with high fibre diets weigh less than those who don't each much fibre. This could be due to the fact that fibre-rich foods are filling. And if you're full you don't feel the need to overeat or snack on treats.

The benefits of fibre (or, to give it its proper name, non-starch polysaccharides) have been known for thousands of years. Hippocrates, known as the father of medicine, advised his wealthy patients to follow the example of their servants and eat brown bread rather than white, 'for its salutary effect on the bowel'. It's recommended that we eat around 18 g of fibre a day, which most of us barely manage because we eat more refined carbohydrates (white, processed foods and sugars) and less fruit and vegetables.

Here's an idea for you ...

Instead of drinking fruit juice, have a litre of water and a couple of oranges. It will save you calories and give you more fibre.

Defining idea …

A game of two halves

There are two kinds of fibre. *Soluble* fibre lowers blood cholesterol levels and slows the absorption of glucose into the blood stream, ensuring there isn't a sudden rise in blood sugar levels – this kind is found particularly in oats and oat bran, barley, brown rice, beans and pulses, and fruit and vegetables. *Insoluble* fibre keeps things moving along in your digestive system, acting a bit like a sponge and soaking up water to expand the bulk of your waste products (poo) – you'll get this kind from eating wheat, wholegrain breads and cereals, corn, green beans, peas and the skins of fruits such as apples.

Everyone knows it's windy

When you increase your fibre consumption, there may be a bit of wind! This is temporary though as you get used to the new foods in your diet. Increasing your activity levels helps as it stimulates the muscles in the torso, helping speedier elimination – you don't want all that waste hanging around.

20. Gum shield

It costs virtually nothing and only takes two minutes a day.

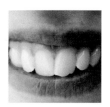

How often do you floss your teeth? Make it every day and it can take almost six and a half years off your real age, believes US anti-ageing guru Dr Michael Roizen. Flossing is the most effective way of staving off gum disease. And gum disease can lead to inflammation of the arteries, a major precursor to heart disease.

Gum disease starts when plaque is left on the gum surface. If it is undisturbed for around a day, the bacteria reproduce and start to become toxic, infecting the gums. These bacteria can be sucked into the lungs, and cross into the bloodstream, triggering inflammation throughout the body – including the arteries.

In its first stages, gum disease is known as gingivitis. The main symptoms are easily bleeding gums and bad breath that disappears when you brush your teeth, but returns shortly afterwards. If ignored, gingivitis can lead to peri-

Here's an idea for you ...

See a dental hygienist at least every six months. They will thoroughly remove all plaque from the gums and under the gumline. Open wide ...

53

Defining idea ...

*'The first thing I do in the morning
is brush my teeth and sharpen my
tongue.'*
DOROTHY PARKER

odontal disease, which is linked with
an increased risk of stroke.

So get your teeth into some good
dental care.

Use an electric toothbrush
Electric toothbrushes are 25% more effective than conventional
brushes at removing plaque. Hold the brush at a 45-degree angle to
the gumline and move the brush back and forth in short strokes.

Floss once a day
When we brush, we tend to reach only the front and back surfaces,
but 90% of gum disease is caused by the bacteria left undisturbed
between the teeth. If you're too tired at night, do it while you're
watching TV or in your car in traffic jams.

Rinse twice a day
Antibacterial mouth rinses dislodge bacteria left behind by brushing.
But don't use one which contains alcohol, as it will dry out the mouth
and encourage the bacteria to breed further.

21. Labelling matters

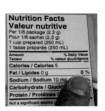

Have you ever looked at the back of a packet of food and wondered where the actual food was?

Food labelling can be hugely confusing. The first rule is that if the ingredient list barely fits on the back of the packet, put it back where you found it. The second rule is that you should recognise the main ingredient: if you don't, or it's something like sugar, reassess your choice.

Beware the sugar monster
Sugar is really one to watch. It wears all sorts of disguises – glucose, fructose, lactose or maltose and, of course, there's always honey. Watch out too for other forms of sugar like sorbitol, xylitol, mannitol and isomalt. The one that's really crept in is the high fructose corn syrups (sugar dextrose), which isn't the same type of sugar as you find in fruit but is extracted from processing cornstarch to yield glucose. It's much cheaper and sweeter than sugar and is, of course, a firm favourite with food manufacturers – sauces, chewing

Here's an idea for you ...

Watch out especially for hydrogenated fats, which may be cunningly listed as 'shortening'. This is particularly found in cakes, biscuits, margarine and ready meals.

Defining idea ...

*'Nothing added, nothing taken away
- that's what we are aiming for!'*
ANON.

gum, fruit drinks, canned fruits, dairy products, jams, sweets, bread, bacon and beer are favourite hiding places. Unfortunately our bodies struggle to use it as effective fuel and it is easily metabolised as fat.

Pass on the salt

Salt (sodium chloride) is added in generous amounts to processed foods and, although you're meant to have a maximum of 6 g a day, you can easily exceed this amount if you don't read the labels. Incidentally, if you're adding a lot of salt to your food, check your nutrient status because you could be short of zinc. A zinc deficiency can stop your taste buds from performing so well.

Butter up

One good bit of news – a little butter probably beats its synthetic cousin margarine if it contains hydrogenated fats. Fats in this form are very similar to Tupperware, molecularly speaking.

22. Games other people play

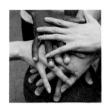

If you left team games behind with teenage crushes, acne and underage drinking, perhaps you're missing out.

There was a problem with the way sports were taught at my school. Those that were any good at it were groomed and encouraged; those who weren't so good were sidelined because the emphasis was always firmly on winning. As an adult, however, you have the option of taking up a sport simply for the pleasure of it. If you take up a new game now, you don't have to be good at it; you simply have to enjoy it. Sports aren't just about fitness either. For many, sport is a means of making new friends or getting away from their normal lives.

Bats
All racquet games are sprint sports that require skill, stamina and explosive strength. They can be great fun and they have a social world all of their own, but to get the most out of

Here's an idea for you ...
Consider Octopush – underwater hockey. No matter how good someone is, their time 'on the ball' ends when they run out of breath.

Defining idea ...

'Any kind of exercise is generally better than no exercise at all.'
ARNOLD SCHWARZENEGGER

them you really need to get fit to play them, rather than play them to get fit. Try getting a coach – or how about badminton? It's about the only racquet game that can truly be played leisurely between like-minded people.

Balls

Ball games like football (soccer) or rugby are also sprint sports, but you can have fun with smaller versions like five-a-side footie or seven-a-side rugby. There are also less-aggressive versions, such as 'touch' rugby too.

Bowls

Bowling isn't the world's most active activity, but it can be applied to different games depending on where you are. Lawn bowling has a more sedate image, and the French game of boules can now be seen on beaches everywhere. The great thing about something like ten-pin bowling is that anyone can have a go and the kit you need will be provided.

23. Not a four-letter word

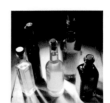

Fat has a bad name, but your body desperately needs it – as long as it's the right sort.

We have a complex about fat. So ingrained is the message of how fat clogs up our arteries, increases our apple-shaped girths, sends our risk of heart disease soaring and is linked to the hooded claw that is cholesterol, that we try to eliminate it from our diets.

However, all fat was not created equal and, as we are finding out to our cost, avoiding all kinds of fat is detrimental to our health.

Oil be damned
Oil in its unprocessed form is highly perishable. It used to be sold fresh door to door and, if not kept cool, would go rancid in a matter of days. Today's polyunsaturated or cholesterol-free oils last longer, but they've

Here's an idea for you ...

Get extra omega-6 from nuts and seeds – and enough omega-3 from oily fish like salmon or sardines (ask at your local healthfood store for veggie alternatives).

Defining idea ...

'May understanding of health be the starship of the next generation. May the worship of disease die with us.'
UDO ERASMUS, oil guru

often been refined very highly using high heat and bleaches that strip them of any nutritional value and may in fact make them unstable and potentially toxic.

Sweet EFA
The chemical building blocks of oils are called fatty acids, and the fatty acids essential to human health (which the body can't manufacture) are called essential fatty acids or EFAs. Without them, we'd be on the fast track to degenerative disease.

EFAs have a more than magical effect on our health. They improve skin and hair condition, aid in the prevention of arthritis, lower cholesterol, protect against heart disease, make your brain work ... in fact, the brain is almost entirely made up of fat, which makes the insult 'fat head' quite a compliment.

Mega Omega
There are two basic groups of EFAs. Omega-6 is found mostly in raw nuts, seeds, legumes and in unsaturated oils such as evening primrose oil or sesame oil; Omega-3 in fresh deep-water fish, some vegetable oils, flaxseed oil and walnut oil.

24. Breathe in, breathe out!

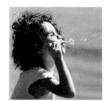

Proper breathing is a forgotten art – and these days we often hold onto our breath out of sheer terror.

It's not called the life breath for nothing. With each breath we exchange carbon dioxide from inside the body with life-giving oxygen from outside. If this incredible process was interrupted for more than a few minutes, it would be curtains.

Breathing is an amazing, miraculous process and it's worked so well that it hasn't changed one iota since we were running away from sabre-toothed beasties. Breathing overrides our in-built, powerful stress responses and slows downs the reaction of the autonomic nervous system. So, the good news is that you have some degree of control over how you react to stress.

Breathing exercises
All you need is a few minutes a day to provide you with a powerful way

Here's an idea for you ...

When you're at the office, why not make your company bathroom your personal breathing booth?

Defining idea ...

of dealing with stress. Here are two exercises, just for starters. Do them!

Exercise 1: observing the breath

Sit on a comfortable chair, your feet on the ground. Close your eyes, rest one hand in your lap and place the other on your tummy. Feel the tummy expand as you breathe in and contract as you breathe out. Breathe in deeply through your nose and silently count 'one'. Breathe out. Breathe in again and count 'two'. Do this for up to 10 breaths and then do it the other way round. Do this for five rounds to start with, building up to 10. Do this once a day.

Exercise 2: anti-stress breath

Try this if you find yourself stressed out and in need of some immediate relief. Breathe in for four counts, hold for four counts and exhale for four counts. Remember to let the out-breath out slowly, not in a rush. Do this for about five cycles, being careful that you don't overdo it otherwise you could end up feeling a bit dizzy.

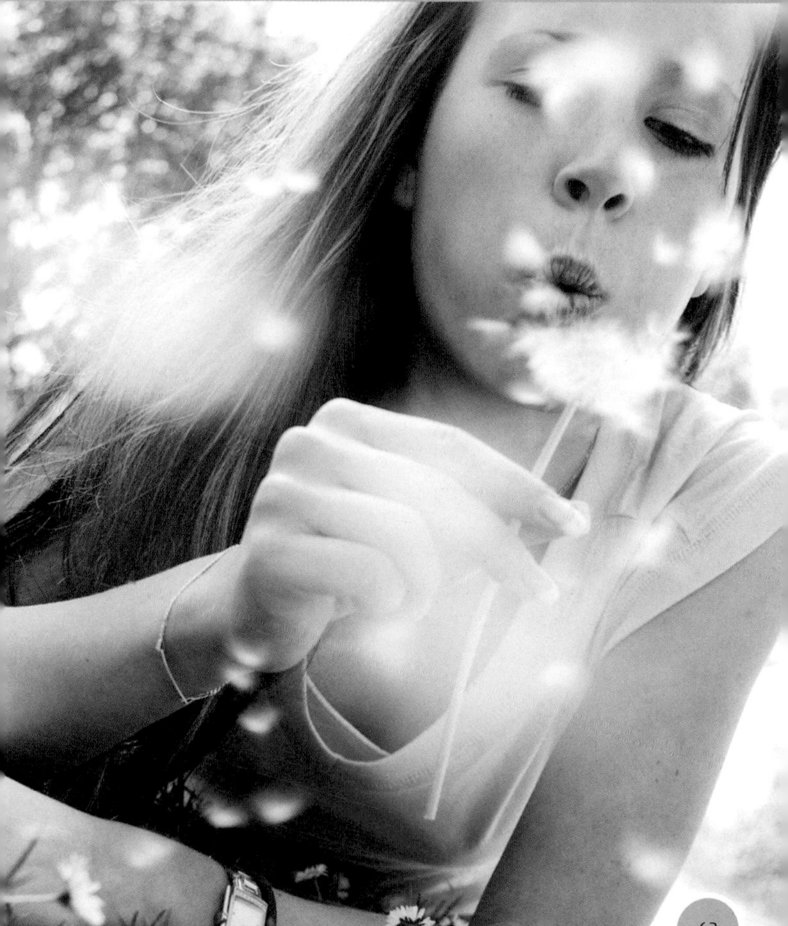

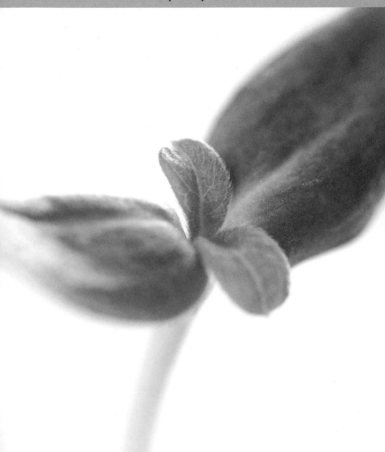

25. New you resolution

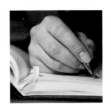

**Don't wait for the next new year.
Keeping fit is a must do – for now!**

Regular physical activity halves the risk of developing heart disease, boosts endorphins and makes you look and feel good – but only if you do it. Resolve to do something small – it doesn't matter what – every day, starting now.

■ Get in the garden and grow your own vegetables.
■ Pick a new hobby you have always dreamed of doing and make it happen.
■ Don't just watch a sport, take part; there are opportunities everywhere.
■ Fidget. Get up and fetch that cup of tea; swing your legs when you're sitting down; or jig around to background music. It all counts.
■ Find a series of exercises that suit you, and do them for five or ten minutes every morning. Choose a sequence that feels right for you.

Here's an idea for you ...

Combine exercise and socialising. Try a regular bike ride with the family, a salsa class or a round of golf with some mates.

Defining idea ...

'The important thing to remember is that this is not a new form of life. It is just a new activity.'
ESTHER DYSON, US journalist

- Monitor your heart rate while you're active. Wear an electronic heart rate monitor on your wrist; go for a waterproof one so you can use it while swimming or exercising in water. Experts recommend that you should exert yourself for twenty to thirty minutes three or more times a week, achieving a heart rate that is at least at 60% but no more than 90% of your maximal heart rate (this varies with age, so ask your doctor or look it up online).

- Join a club. You don't have to go to a gym or play sports or use special equipment, but you'll get lots of activity done this way.

- Take advantage of the personal trainer or coach at your gym or club. If you've got a training plan and someone monitoring your progress you'll go far.

- Choose the right shoes and clothes for your activity so you can walk, run and move without doing yourself harm.

26. Train your private army

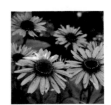

A strong immune system fights off invasion by foreign organisms that lead to disease. Here's how to keep your troops in peak condition.

Every day, hordes of bugs try to get inside your body. Luckily the body has an army of scavenging white blood cells, looking for invaders. If a scavenging cell spots one, it's transported to the nearest lymph glands and destroyed before it's even had a chance to wave a white flag.

Three main factors that lead to weak links in your inner defences:

What you eat
Your immune system works best with a full range of vitamins and minerals. But even people who eat a balanced diet often show deficiencies: with today's sedentary lifestyle, we may not

Here's an idea for you ...

Regular massage can boost the immune system by increasing levels of infection-fighting cells. Simply get a tennis ball, lean against a wall and roll the ball around between your back and shoulders and the wall.

Defining idea …

'Hope, purpose and determination have electrochemical connections that affect the immune system.'
NORMAN COUSINS, writer

be able to eat enough to get the full range of micronutrients we need; and intensive farming and food processing deplete food of micronutrients. Take a good supplement every day.

Your environment

If you bombard your body with extra invaders on a regular basis, the effectiveness of T-cells (your special forces) is weakened and disease-causing bugs multiply. While you can't control the many bacteria and viruses that assault you every day, you can control additional toxic invaders such as cigarette smoke and, to a lesser extent, environmental pollution.

The mind/body factor

Undergoing regular stress is like offering a personal invitation to foreign invaders to walk through the chinks in your armour. People in one study were most likely to develop a cold if they had experienced a negative life event in the past year. Relax: your troops will be stronger for it.

27. The sex factor

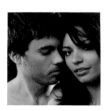

People who have frequent sex live longer. Here's how to put the passion back into your life.

Sex is good for you. Hurrah! It improves cholesterol levels, increasing circulation and releasing endorphins, but it may also release chemicals that benefit the immune system. Frequent ejaculations in men may reduce the risk of prostate cancer by as much as 33%.

A healthy sex life can keep you looking young too. One study of 3500 people who looked on average ten years younger than their real age found that most were making love around three times a week (the average is around once a week).

It seems straightforward enough – have more sex if you want to live longer. Except that it's not just something you can simply add to the bottom of your daily 'to do' list ('ring accountant, sort out the shed, defrost supper, have a shag').

Here's an idea for you ...

Fancy playing? If you really can't face going to a sex shop, or there isn't one near you, check out websites like www.coco-de-mer.co.uk.

69

Defining idea ...

One of the main reasons we go off sex with our long-term partners is because there are so many distractions in life – paying the bills, doing the washing up, dealing with each other's families and the kids. Sex arises out of the quality of a relationship as a whole. To prioritise your sex life, you have to strengthen the whole relationship. So forget the dishes, leave the answerphone on and sit down to pay each other some real attention. Make time to have a glass of wine and a chat together. Don't just talk practicalities, talk about your hopes and dreams. And make each other laugh!

Then put a little imagination into trying something new. It doesn't need to be super-kinky – something as simple as scented massage oil and candlelight can work wonders. Experimenting is the best way of finding out what works for both of you. Now, when has homework ever been as much fun?

28. Pump some iron

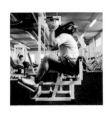

Lifting weights isn't just for bodybuilders. Strength training is insurance for any body.

The only proven way to boost your metabolic rate is to build lean muscle tissue by regular strength training. A strength-training exercise is simply any exercise that puts your muscles under tension, which can be done using your own body weight. You don't have to go to a gym or wear exercise gear. Grunting isn't obligatory, either!

Your mini workout
Aim to do this at least once a week. Warm up first with five minutes of marching on the spot, and do some stretches at the end.

1 *Squats with side lift.* Stand with your feet slightly more than hip-width apart. Lower your bottom, hold for one breath then push yourself back up, raising your right leg out to the side as you do. Repeating with the left leg.

Here's an idea for you ...

Do open-door press-ups while you're waiting for the kettle. With hands just below shoulder-height on either side of an open door frame, raise up on your toes then bend your arms at the elbows and push back. Repeat till it boils!

Defining idea ...

'Inward calm cannot be maintained unless physical strength is replenished.'
Buddhist philosophy

2   *Leg lunges.* Stand with your feet slightly more than hip-width apart. Take a large step backwards with your right leg. Lower your right knee to the floor, bending your left leg as you do. Go as low as you can before pushing off and returning to the start. Repeat with your left leg.

3   *Press-ups.* Start on your hands and knees, with your hands facing forward and in line with your shoulders, at a half-body-width distance from your body, your knees behind your body, your back straight. Push down until you almost reach the floor then push back up. Keep your abs tight the whole time.

4   *Front raises.* Stand with your legs slightly more than hip-width apart, and knees 'soft'. Hold weights or water bottles by the sides of your body, palms downwards. Slowly raise your arms, keeping them straight, until they are at chest height. Repeat.

29. Water, baby

What's to know about water? Even with this simple liquid, there are health choices to be made.

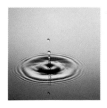

On tap or on the bottle?
Most tap water will contain a cocktail of contaminates, most commonly lead, aluminium and pesticides – but bottled water isn't necessarily the purest.

With bottles, water can be labelled mineral, spring or table water. Mineral water is generally from a pure, underground source, where the rocks and earth have naturally filtered it. Spring water also comes from a filtered underground source, but does not have to be bottled on the spot. Table water is definitely the dodgiest dude: it could include tap water, so you could just be wasting your money. Watch out for artificially carbonated table and spring water as this can rob the vital minerals in the body by binding to them. Also, look at the proportion of minerals – remember that salt (sodium) will dehydrate the body slightly.

Here's an idea for you …

If you're not used to drinking masses of water, increase your intake slowly by just one ½-litre bottle a day at first.

Defining idea ...

'Water, water, everywhere,
Nor any drop to drink.'
SAMUEL TAYLOR COLERIDGE, *The Rime of the Ancient Mariner*

Fishy business

Every now and then, there'll be a TV programme featuring male fish turning into female fish. Scare stories aside, the point is that we're being continuously exposed to xeno-oestrogens (foreign oestrogens) in our environment and these can have a feminising effect on our bodies. One source of these foreign oestrogens is through plastics – so don't leave your water in the sun in a plastic bottle.

Water works

What are the best choices then? Well, one cheap solution is to get a filter jug, which removes the bug-busting chlorine element. The carbon filter takes out some minerals, so change it at regular intervals to prevent manky old ones from leaching bacteria back in. You could have a filter attached to your tap, or consider the more expensive, but definitely superior, reverse osmosis systems which separate the water from the other elements that are contained in it (NASA developed this for its astronauts).

30. Game for a laugh

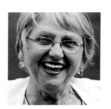

Laughter reduces stress, lowers blood pressure, relieves pain, oxygenates the blood and strengthens the immune system. Funny, eh?

Two hunters are out in the woods when one of them collapses. The other guy whips out his phone and calls the emergency services: 'My friend is dead! What can I do?' The operator says 'Calm down, I can help. First, let's make sure he's dead.' There is a silence, then a shot is heard. The guy says to the operator: 'OK, now what?'

That is officially the world's funniest joke – and if you laughed when you read it, you've given your immune system a huge boost. Researchers have shown that laughter reduces the levels of the stress hormones cortisone and adrenaline and boosts your number of infection-fighting white T-cells.

During laughter, blood pressure rises; after, it drops a point lower than be-fore. Laughter may even improve your

Here's an idea for you ...

Moving your face into a smile makes your brain release happy-chemicals, making you feel like smiling even more. And it takes half as many muscles to smile as it does to frown.

'One laugh is worth two tablets.'
FREDDIE FRANKL, psychiatrist

physical fitness. Have a real belly laugh and around 400 muscles of your body will move – it's like internal aerobics. If you could keep up a belly laugh for a full hour, you could even laugh off as many as 500 calories.

The problem is that the older we get, the more it takes to make us laugh. At 4 we laugh 400 times a day. By age 30, it's down to around 15. A small child doesn't need searing political satire to raise a smile. They'll laugh at any noise that vaguely resembles passing wind. When did we lose this sense of fun?

Deciding to laugh more every day sounds like a simple way to live longer, but it's easier said than done. Polish up a rusty sense of humour with some Simpsons DVDs. Swap jokes by email. Or hang out with some small kids.

31. Get hooked on fish

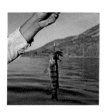

Your grandmother was talking sense after all – fish really is good for your brain and a daily dose of cod liver oil will keep you strong and healthy.

Fish help you look and feel younger. It all comes down to some special fatty acids found in fish called omega-3s. These oils are vital for the functioning of every cell in our bodies, and yet our bodies cannot make them – we have to get them from food. Two particularly valuable omega-3s are docosahexaenoic acid (DHA) and eicosapentanoic acid (EPA) and you'll find high levels in salmon, herrings, sardines, pilchards, mackerel, tuna and trout. A recent best-selling book even recommended eating salmon three times a day instead of having a facelift.

Inuit all along

Did you know the Inuit don't have a word in their language for heart attack because it's so rare among them? This is thought to be thanks to their diet – but if you don't fancy whale or seal blubber all winter, don't worry: you get the same benefits from eating the fish whales and seals eat: salmon, herring, anchovies, mackerel

Here's an idea for you …

Tins are also good. Add a tin of anchovies to tomato-based pasta sauces or use as a pizza topping. Or mash a tin of sardines, herring or pilchards onto multigrain toast.

Defining idea ...

'Fish, to taste good, must swim three times: in water, in butter and in wine.'
Polish proverb

and tuna. The omega-3 fatty acids 'calm down' the artery walls, as well as reducing production of bad LDL cholesterol, raising levels of good HDL cholesterol, lowering blood pressure and reducing irregular heart beats.

Thanks to realms of other studies, we now know that these valuable oils play a role in staving off stroke and breast cancer, fighting asthma and protecting joints. There's scientific research to back up what our ancestors knew by instinct – that fish is good for the brain. One study found that older people who eat fish or seafood once a week have a significantly lower risk of developing dementia.

Omega-3s work best as part of a double act with another group of essential oils called omega-6s, found in vegetable oils such as sunflower, soy, hemp and linseed, which are important for lowering blood cholesterol and supporting the skin. Thanks to the widespread use of sunflower oil in food processing, few of us are deficient in omega-6s, but at the same time, intake of omega-3s has dropped by more than half (we don't eat so much fish and tend to go for low fat varieties such as cod and haddock rather than herring and mackerel). Scientists now believe that too many omega-6s in the diet can undo the good work of omega-3s. To redress the balance, try to cut down on fried and processed foods and margarines and eat more oily fish – aim for a minimum of twice a week.

32. Skin from within

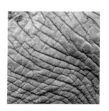

With great nutrition and a little care, you can achieve great-looking skin in no time at all.

Healthy skin is part of a healthy body, and changes the face you present to the world too. Here are some simple steps to looking after your body's biggest organ.

Tutti frutti

You probably don't need me to tell you that fruit and vegetables are the main ingredients for healthy, youthful skin. The vitamins and minerals they contain perform an antioxidant function, mopping up reactions caused by free radicals (unstable molecules created by such things as stress, pollution and certain foods). Free radicals can ultimately cause degenerative diseases such as cancer and heart disease, not to mention premature ageing (where your skin comes in).

Here's an idea for you ...

Try to eat at least five portions of fruit and vegetables daily. And the more colours the better – try red peppers, yellow peppers, green peppers, red cabbage, sweet potatoes, etc. This way you can get enough antioxidants to help counter the effects of pollution. Be sure to buy organic though, as otherwise you could add to your toxic load!

Defining idea …

'All the beauty in the world, 'tis but skin deep.'
RALPH VENNING

Berries and fruits and vegetables with red, purple and blue colouring are particularly good because they're stuffed with antioxidants and contain a group of flavonoids called anthocyanidins, thought to be much more powerful than vitamin E.

Water your face daily

Drinking pure, fresh water flushes toxins through your system and hydrates cells carrying essential nutrients to every part of your body. I probably didn't need to tell you that either. Aim to drink about 2 litres (3.5 pints) daily. Don't overdo it though or you could end up flushing minerals out of your system, especially if you're gulping rather than sipping.

Fat face

The other essential ingredient to healthy skin is fat. Not any old fat, but essential fatty acids (EFAs), especially Omega-3. EFAs work as a kind of waterproofer because they stop fluids escaping from your body's cells, keeping it plumped up and moisturised. Take a good quality fish oil supplement for three months (or flaxseed if you're vegetarian) and note the quality of skin on the back of your hands. You should also decrease the amount of saturated and processed fats in your diet, as these compete, making the job of the good more difficult.

33. Yoga

Yoga is about being rather than doing. It's non-competitive and a great balancer for the type of exercise you might do at the gym.

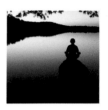

Not so long ago, if you admitted you did yoga you'd have been classed as a New Age weirdo and given a wide berth. Today, if you're not into yoga you're the weird one. So, get with the programme!

In essence, all types of yoga are about using the body and breathing to help calm the mind in order to produce a feeling of wellbeing. Yoga is a great stress buster and it's easy to do at any age so it's never too late to start. Flexibility is a vital component, both physical and mental – a flexible mind equals a flexible body. Yoga generally uses asanas (postures) that usually retain their ancient names: the fish, the bridge, the bow, the scorpion, etc. They are believed to bring benefits to different areas of the body and are held for a period of time to stretch and strengthen muscles. Worth a try? The simplest asana is the corpse position, which involves lying down

Here's an idea for you ...

Yoga has evolved to incorporate quite a few different types. Check out www.yogapoint.com. You might want to experiment by going to a few classes.

Defining idea ...

on your back on the floor with your eyes closed. Your breathing should be slow and steady, and your arms should be held at a 45-degree angle away from the body.

Yoga incorporates ideas of a 'proper' diet too. This is vegetarian, comprising Sattic foods such as wholemeal grains and fresh fruit and vegetables. Diet as a whole is divided up into three main sections: Sattic foods, which I've already mentioned; Rajasic foods, which are hot and bitter foods (e.g. coffee, tea, chocolate, salt, strong herbs, fish) that are considered to destroy the mind–body equilibrium; and Tamasic foods (e.g. meat, alcohol, garlic, onions), which neither benefit the mind nor the body as they encourage a sense of inertia.

34. Superfoods

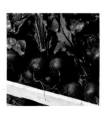

In their own small way, superfoods can be your own personal superheroes.

Most fruit and vegetables are, of course, superfoods – a kiwi, for example, contains twice as much vitamin C than an orange. And pineapples have both an antibiotic and anti-inflammatory effect – so where should we start? With your ABC, of course.

A is for …

Apples are a number one superfood. Packed with vitamin C, apples also boast pectin, which helps keep cholesterol levels stable and protects us from pollution. On top of all this, the malic and tartaric acid in apples help neutralise the acid by-products of indigestion and help your body cope with dietary excesses.

B is for …

Beetroot was used in Romany medi-cine as a blood-builder for patients that looked pale and run down. Don't overdo it though, as beetroot

Here's an idea for you …

Consider taking superfoods in powder form – you can get a day's worth of vegetable requirements in one drink. Check out www.kiki-health.com.

Defining idea ...

'If you could plant one tree in your garden, it should be an apple tree.'
MAURICE MESSEGUE, herbalist

is such a powerful detoxicant that too much could be a strain on your system. Broccoli is another big super hero. It has been demonstrated in a number of studies to have a protective effect against cancer. And yet another superfood is the humble carrot.

C is for ...
A single carrot supplies a whole day's vitamin A requirements and helps protect you against cancer. Add ginger to carrot juice to fend off colds and flu, or as a remedy against sickness and nausea. Or blood-purifying parsley which is bursting with manganese, iron, copper, calcium, phosphorous, sodium, potassium and magnesium.

Squeeze me!
So how can you obtain the amazing health benefits from superfoods? Juice it. Juice is easy to assimilate and is completely natural. Juice will give you access to enzymes to aid digestion, brain stimulation and cellular energy; phytochemicals, which are linked with disease-busting properties; and nutrients, which juice you up with energy!

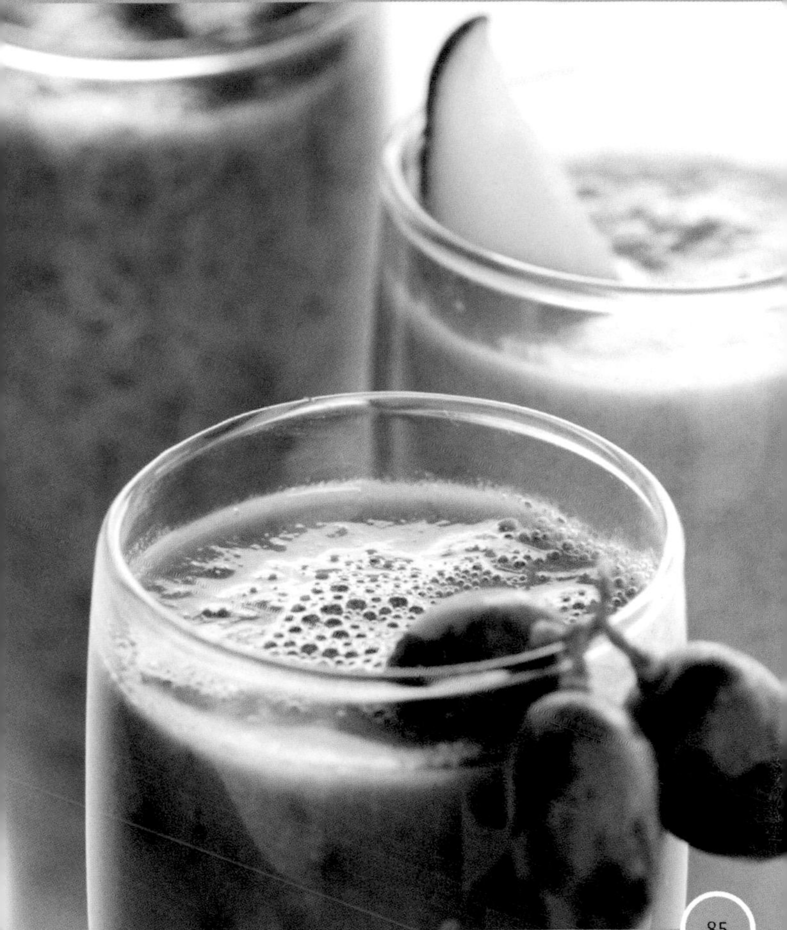

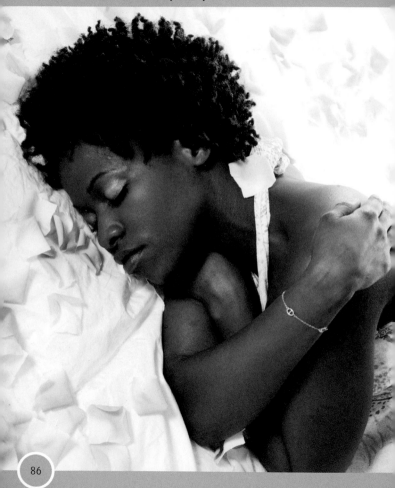

35. The sleep solution

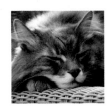

Ever looked in the mirror after a late night and thought you looked older? It's not your imagination.

If you cut back on sleep, you're cutting back on growth hormone and giving your body less chance to repair itself. The ideal amount is between six and eight hours. Get less than this and you start to build up a sleep debt and that's bad news. One study found that women who got five hours of sleep or less nightly over a decade had a 39% greater risk of heart attack than those who managed eight hours.

But it's not just growth hormone doing wonders while you sleep. Recently scientists discovered that melatonin, the 'dark hormone' that triggers sleep, is a potent antioxidant. It's thought to be as effective as vitamins C and E as it gets right inside your body's cells where it guards against DNA damage.

Here's an idea for you ...

Try to go to bed and get up at the same time each day – even at weekends. If you still feel tired during the day, push your bedtime back by fifteen minutes a week until you wake up feeling refreshed.

Defining idea ...

We tend to take sleep for granted
– and just expect it to happen. But
what we do through the day has a
direct effect on how we sleep at night.
Ideally, avoid caffeine from lunchtime
onwards: it can remain in the body
for hours. Restrict alcohol to one or two small glasses of wine early
evening and avoid eating a large meal later than three hours before
you intend to go to bed – this increases your metabolic rate.

Temperature and light need to be right too. Try having a warm bath
before bed – studies have shown that a drop in body temperature
triggers the brain's sleep response – and keep your bedroom cool.

Then try wearing a mask at night (especially in summer) and expos-
ing yourself to bright light as soon as you wake up.

36. The 'big C'

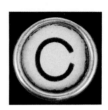

Cancer is a scary word, but more than 90% of cancers are preventable.

Fewer than 10% of all cancers are linked to genetic inheritance. The rest are linked to lifestyle – something you have control over. But to fight your enemy, you must know it, so here's a simple-to-understand guide to why cancer happens – and what you can do to reduce the risk.

Cancer begins with just one cell that suddenly begins growing and dividing again until it forms a tumour. If it becomes large enough or spreads, it can prevent the body's organs from working efficiently, which, if left unchecked, can be fatal.

Most of the body (99%) is made up of cells that continually grow, divide and then die. When each cell divides, it copies its DNA into the new cell. Problems begin when a mistake is made in the duplication process, or when the DNA is damaged. In both

Here's an idea for you ...

Pucker up! Did you know that wearing lipstick reduces the risk of lip cancer by 50%? Men, don't miss out – use protective lip salve.

Defining idea …

'Since I came to the White House, I got two hearing aids, a colon operation, skin cancer, a prostate operation and I was shot. The damn thing is I've never felt better in my life.'
RONALD REAGAN

cases, a mutation occurs which is then passed on when a cell divides. Just sometimes, a certain type of mutation tells the cell to begin growing and dividing uncontrollably.

At this point, a strong immune system will remove the destructive cells – but experts believe that cancer occurs when we're older because the immune system is simply less efficient. Which is good news – because there's much you can do to prevent the ageing of the immune system. Eating a diet high in fruit and vegetables is one of the easiest and most effective ways of doing this.

At the risk of stating the glaringly obvious, prevention is better than cure. So avoid the known cancer-causing factors such as smoking, obesity and poor nutrition too. Now, what's scary about that?

37. Pet theories

They can raise your spirits, provide you with love and regular exercise – and demand very little in return. Get a pet!

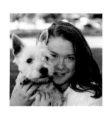

Walkies!

You make resolutions to exercise regularly. But it's hard to do it for yourself when it's cold and wet or you're ultra-tired or just too busy. But if you've got a dog, one look at those soulful, begging eyes and off you go. Once, twice a day, you'll soon do all the walking you're supposed to. You might take your pet along for company, or even for protection from muggers, while you run or cycle. Going up the size scale, keeping a horse will give you a different kind of regular exercise, unless you pay others to train and ride it for racing and other track competitions. Dreaming of riding with the wind in your face, being at one with your animal, will keep you going through gruelling days at work, too.

There, there

Pets bring you other benefits too. Stroking a cat, for example, can help

Here's an idea for you …

If you don't fancy having a pet of your own, consider pet-sitting as an occasional job. Homes for abandoned dogs are often looking for volunteer walkers, too.

Defining idea ...

'Animals are such agreeable friends – they ask no questions, they pass no criticisms.'
GEORGE ELIOT

you relax, and caring for an animal can help you climb out of a low mental state. Your pet will give you something else to think about. You can chat to your pet budgie or rat and tell them your problems without being judged or interrupted. Having a cat or dog to come home to means there's always someone pleased to see you too. And if you invest attention and love in them, they regard you as being the centre of their world.

Hoovering up

Finally, you'll be more inclined to trim the fat off food or cut down what you eat if you to give what's left over to your dog or pet rat or whatever, rather than chuck it in the bin. So your pet will, indirectly, even encourage you to eat more healthily.

38. Get organic

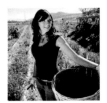

We're turning to organic food in our droves. But is it worth it?

Apart from avoiding everything from pesticide residue in pears to mercury poisoning from tuna, people are buying organic because of the taste. Remember how tomatoes should taste? Like organic ones.

Chemical dependency
The drive to increase productivity means that many non-organic fruit and vegetables contain weedkillers, pesticides and fertilizers. Fruit and vegetables have to look perfect for supermarkets too. But what effects do these chemicals have on human health? Potentially anxiety, hyperactivity, digestive problems and muscle weakness.

Meat madness
The biggest worries come in the form of intensively farmed meat products: crazy cows, potty pigs – it's no joke. It's just not possible to crowd animals into such tight spaces without using industrial strength pesticides to stop disease spreading.

Here's an idea for you ...

Prioritise. Go organic first with fruit and veg you'd normally peel. Then opt for organic milk and beef: 'normal' cows are treated with growth promoters.

93

Defining idea ...

'Organic farming delivers the highest quality, best-tasting food, while helping to maintain the landscape and rural communities.'
PRINCE CHARLES

A time and a place
To get the best organic fruit and vegetables, eat what's local and in season. If it's produced abroad, vitamins and mineral content are lost on the journey here.

Don't be had
Remember that just because it says its organic on the packet, it doesn't mean that it's better for you. Once organic products have been turned into a crisp, cake or biscuit, for example, you'll have more or less the same concerns as with the conventional versions: high sugar and fat.

Expect the inspection
Farmers need a licence to legally use the term 'organic'. They must follow guidelines on how to produce food to organic standards and they're inspected regularly. Visit www.soilassociation.org to find out more.

How?
Look in your supermarket for the organic section, try the healthfood shop, or see if you can have a box delivered to your door (try the web to find a company that suits your needs).

39. On the level

Some numbers are luckier than others ... like anything below 5, for your cholesterol level.

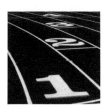

Cholesterol plays a vital role in the formation of cell walls and some of the body's essential chemicals, including some hormones. And most cholesterol is in fact made by the body itself. So what's all the fuss about, you ask? Simple. Too much cholesterol is a major risk factor for heart disease – and an estimated seven out of ten people over the age of 45 have too much.

You can get your cholesterol measured by your doctor, and you'll be given a figure. Well, three, in fact. You'll be given a total cholesterol reading (ideally this should be lower than 5), but also a ratio of your LDL to HDL cholesterol (ideally, 3 to 1).

Cholesterol uses the blood as its road system, riding on vehicles made up of proteins. On its journey from the liver to the cells that need it, it rides in low density lipoproteins (LDL). Any cholesterol that's not needed is

Here's an idea for you ...

If you've never had your cholesterol checked, call your doctor now and make an appointment. All the test involves is a pinprick of blood from a finger.

Defining idea ...

'It is a scientific fact that your body
will not absorb cholesterol if you take
it from another person's plate.'
DAVE BARRY, US humorist

returned to the liver on HDL or high
density lipoproteins. The trouble begins when there is too much LDL and
not enough HDL. The excess amounts
of cholesterol are simply dumped on
the artery walls.

So your aim is to lower your LDL cholesterol and boost your HDL.
And one of the easiest ways to do this is to eat more fat – of the right
kind. Fish oil works wonders. Try a tin of sardines in tomato sauce,
mashed up with a squirt of lemon juice, on a slice of toast – delicious!
And monounsaturated fats are also good too – found in high quantities in olive oil, rapeseed oil, linseed, nuts and avocados. Switch to
olive oil for frying and dressings.

40. Take a walk on the wild side

Get a bit of perspective on life, while getting yourself in peak condition too.

Walking can mean more than popping out to the corner shop for twenty Marlboro. Why not take a chance on adventure walking? A special weekend in the country once or twice a year will inspire you for the everyday stuff like walking to work.

Make sure you're fully prepared first. Get kitted out with the right gear before you set out.

Equipment for your own miracle
In this country, great wet-weather gear is a must. I'm not talking fisherman's yellow galoshes and capes – these days you can get very light wet-weather gear that will fold up and fit into you pocket. Don't just get the top; invest in the trousers as well – you'll be glad

Here's an idea for you ...

Take a holiday that includes guided walks in wonderful countryside. Try www.atg-oxford.co.uk, www.walkworldwide.com or www.theultimatetravelcompany.co.uk.

97

Defining idea …

'You cannot teach a crab to walk in a straight line.'
ARISTOPHENES

you did one long, rainy, windswept day.

Next, track down the right boots. The boots need to be protective of the ankles, waterproof, not too heavy and to have a good grip. Remember that you could well have thick socks to allow for so don't buy them too small. Oh, and get proper walking socks too. A good outdoor shop should be able to advise you.

The other essential piece of kit is your rucksack. Choose one with a middle strap to protect your back, and loads of pockets, then pack some basic survival gear. You'll need matches (in a little plastic bag), a Swiss army knife, a foil blanket, a water bottle. oatcakes, nuts and maybe some dark chocolate (temperature permitting). Add a whistle just in case you need to attract attention, a hat, good sunglasses and some sunscreen. A map is good, as long as you can read it. And you'll need to carry at least a litre of water.

Don't forget to pack a small medical kit that includes some rehydration sachets (electrolyte formulas) and some plasters for those pesky blisters.

41. Stay stopped

Nicotine is always waiting round the next corner, so you need to keep reminding yourself why and how you gave up.

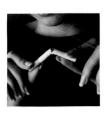

If you've given up smoking but fear you might slip, don't panic. First, remember why you gave up smoking in the first place. Because you wanted to. Then read on …

More than a match
Life is made up of patterns, and humans love to tread those comforting, familiar paths. What you must do more than anything is disrupt those patterns that trigger the desire to smoke. Get rid of all the smoking paraphernalia that litters your life. Change the ways you do things, especially anything that you can connect to smoking – where you sit, how you use the telephone, what order you do things in.

Break up the smoking pattern; create a new non-smoking one in its place.

Here's an idea for you …

Write down all the reasons why you gave up smoking in the first place. The put it somewhere you'll see it every day.

Defining idea …

'I'll go to a club [in Britain], but you guys smoke so friggin' much, I can't sing for ages after. If everyone in England stops smoking cigarettes then I'll come and party.'
MARIAH CAREY, singer

You've got a friend in me
Support is a vital ingredient in the recipe for success. A 'quit smoking' group, friends, colleagues at work, but particularly members of your family, can provide the extra discipline and morale boosts to keep you on the straight and narrow.

Walk the walk
Prove to everyone you're bigger than the habit. Celebrate each new day, the increased money, the improved health. Live to 100 and patronise the other 'mere' pensioners.

One day at a time
You're a smoker, even when you've stopped. It's a bit like being an alcoholic. Be strong every day. Resist. Remember one cigarette is never going to be enough; it'll be the first of many, the first of thousands. Promise yourself you'll never, ever start again.

42. Supplementary benefits

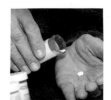

Most nutritionists believe everyone benefits from taking a good daily supplement. But what's 'good'?

Tricky. It's not simply a case of 'more is better' – your body (and your bank balance) will thank you for making an informed choice of a select few. Here's a simple four-step guide to successfully negotiating the supplement maze.

1 *Start with a daily multivitamin/mineral supplement.* Look for one that includes selenium – one study found that 100 mcg of selenium taken daily reduced the death rate among cancer patients. Ideally, it should also include around 50 mg of magnesium, which helps to lower blood pressure.

2 *Boost your vitamin C.* Vitamin C's main job is to eliminate free radicals looking to damage your DNA. When it has a spare moment, it also helps heal artery walls, reduce cholesterol, lower blood pressure

Here's an idea for you ...

Nutritionists say it doesn't matter what time of day you take your vitamins, as long as they're taken at roughly the same time every day. Keep your bottles next to the kettle as a reminder!

Defining idea …

'Every human being is the author of his own health or disease.'
THE BUDDHA

and fight cancer. Make sure you eat some citrus food every day, with a supplement of up to 1000 mg – the current recommended safe upper limit.

3   *Boost your vitamin E.* Vitamin E can lower the risk of heart attack in women by as much as 40% and in men by 35%. If vitamin E is given to people who already show signs of heart disease, it can reduce the risk of heart attack by as much as 75%. In an ideal world, vitamin E likes to work with vitamin C. Eat wholegrain cereals, bread, rice or pasta plus green leafy vegetables every day, supplemented with up to 540 mg.

4   *Boost your Bs.* Homocysteine is an amino acid, and scientists are linking high homocysteine levels with a higher risk of heart disease. Just take a supplement of 400 mcg of folic acid every day, as part of a B complex supplement, and you'll substantially reduce your homocysteine to safe levels.

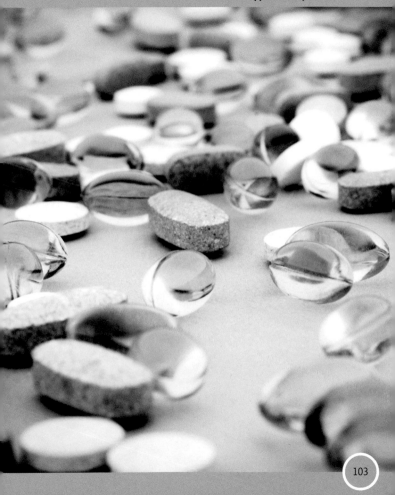

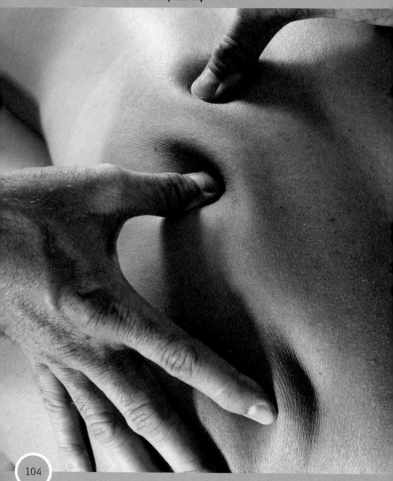

43. Ooh, that feels good!

The sense of touch is a wonderful thing. Comforting, reassuring, arousing – but there's a time and place for everything.

If you've had a massage, then you'll know just how good it can feel – even the most vigorous are eventually deeply satisfying, unless your therapist is overenthusiastic and accidentally debones you in the tenderising process. Just joking. A good massage is very, very, and sometimes very, relaxing. In fact, a number of studies have shown that massage therapy can seriously decrease physical and mental stress.

If you've not yet experienced the pleasure, and sometimes pain, of a good massage, then you may be a little anxious. That's understandable. You've not had one before, so it's very likely that your understanding of the whole process is based largely on urban myth rather than fact. Locker room or ladies' room talk usually revolves around Baywatch-esque therapists who will go to any length to satisfy your wildest dreams. Plus, of course, it depends which country

Defining idea ...

'How beautiful it is to do nothing, and then rest afterward.'
Spanish proverb

you are in. Just as different countries have different cultural behaviours, so they also have different expectations and techniques when practising massage. When it comes down to the nitty-gritty though, once the excitement of these fantasies has past and someone has decided to give it a go, the question that is at the forefront of their mind is not how much will it cost and what do I get for that, but how much clothing do I need to remove?

Relax. Any genuine massage therapist has dealt with the same concerns many times before – and seen a host of different body shapes and sizes. If you feel uncomfortable, ask what's expected. And if you still feel uncomfortable, tell them what you are comfortable with. Go for a head massage, or just your neck and shoulders. If you like it, you can choose to try more next time you book in.

44. Tall orders

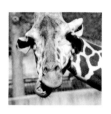

Perfect posture could be your short cut to a leaner, longer shape and a fitter, happier you.

Good posture works wonders. It improves your breathing, digestion and circulation, helps your bones and makes you look like you're brimming with health and confidence.

Try this: Sit up straight for five minutes with your head up and shoulders dropped. Concentrate on your breathing. How do you feel? Relaxed? Of course you do! So, where can you take it next?

Pilates
Pilates is a re-education programme for your muscles, which are used to a lifetime of abuse. It aims, through often very subtle movements, to correct these bad habits. One of the major features is core stability but it can be hard to 'get' without a teacher. Try your gym: one-to-one tuition can be expensive.

Here's an idea for you ...

Experiment with DVDs of your new fads. If you enjoy doing a particular discipline at home, you can move on to classes knowing you'll like them.

Defining idea ...

'*Never grow a wishbone, daughter,
where your backbone ought to be.*'
**CLEMENTINE PADDLEFORD,
author**

Alexander technique

Think how easily small kids move. However, as we grow older and tense up our posture suffers, often resulting in migraine, arthritis, neck pain and back pain. The Alexander Technique tries to correct over-tensed muscles, particularly looking at how the head relates to the spine. It's often taught privately so prepare yourself for an investment. Check out www.alexandertechnique.com.

Just be with t'ai chi

T'ai chi is a slow-moving choreography – each minute movement shifts the body's weight subtly from one leg to the other. Practiced properly, flexibility, balance and strength are all within your grasp. Look for t'ai chi advertised locally. Again, many gyms now run classes. Be warned, t'ai chi is a lifelong journey, not something you master overnight.

Don't want to do the work?

What about getting a chiropractor, osteopath or physiotherapist to help fix your posture? A chiropractor is concerned with your spine; osteopathic treatment concentrates on the relationships within the structure of the body; and physiotherapists can assess your posture then give you exercises to do.

45. To beef or not to beef?

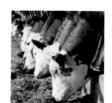

Vegetarians live longer and suffer less heart disease and cancer. Is it time to ditch the meat?

You can look forward to ten extra years of disease-free living than meat-eaters and you're 39% less likely to die from cancer. You're also 30% less likely to die of heart disease. Dr Colin Campbell, chairman of the World Cancer Research Fund, believes that 'the vast majority, perhaps 80 to 90%, of all cancers, cardiovascular diseases and other forms of degenerative illness can be prevented, at least until very old age, simply by adopting a plant-based diet'.

But hang on, you're thinking, if we're designed to munch plants, how come our cavemen ancestors ate meat? It's a good point. Trouble is, although the human race did evolve as omnivores, we now eat more meat in a week than our ancestors did in months.

And most meat-eaters also eat too much protein. According to the World

Here's an idea for you ..

Eat your beans. Pulses are not only a good source of protein – they're also high in disease-fighting antioxidants.

Defining idea …

'It always seems to me that man was not born to be a carnivore.'
ALBERT EINSTEIN

Health Organisation, we need around 35 g of protein a day, but the average meat-eating woman eats around 65 g and the average man, 90 g.

But what if you're a diehard meat fan who can't bear the thought of life without a Sunday roast? Don't despair – omnivores who eat above average amounts of fruit and vegetables can cut their risk of most cancers by 50–75%. And by increasing the amount of plant foods you eat, you'll probably find you naturally cut back on meat consumption.

It's a myth that meat is the best source of protein – it's also found in some surprising foods, like brown rice for instance. Add a small tin of mixed beans (rinse them in a sieve under the tap first) to cooked, cooled brown rice and sprinkle with a few drops of sesame oil to taste. Garnish with fresh coriander. Who needs meat?

46. Run? With my reputation?

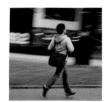

Right now, running for the bus could be only a dream. But find your own perfect pace and you'll never look back.

It's relatively cheap. Anyone can do it pretty much anywhere. It's still about the best calorie-burning exercise known to man and it builds up bone density, endurance, toned thighs and stronger heart and lungs. And it can be a special time, a quiet time set aside for thinking things over or perhaps not thinking things over. So, what's holding you back?

For many, it's the fear that we just can't do it. So, take it one step at a time (so to speak). Start by running for a minute, walking for a minute, for a total of five or ten minutes. Gradually build up the running time, while keeping the walking time the same, and raise the total to fifteen, twenty, twenty five minutes. And whenever you feel comfortable,

Here's an idea for you ...

Having a running partner can make all the difference. It can make time fly and help motivate you. Ask a mate or join a club.

Defining idea ...

'You really just can't beat the outdoors. You get to see other runners and there's always somewhere to spit.'
DRAGON BREATH, one of the runners in the Runners World online community.

reduce the walking time to 30 seconds. Before you know, it you'll be running farther than you ever thought possible.

Plan where you will run. Take enough money to buy a bus ticket back in case you get tired or sprain something. Know where you are going and where you will find water, such as a drinking fountain, a café or from a bottle you take with you. Try not to have to cross roads (it's easy for your attention to wander at crucial moments) or run past potential stress factors such as a corner where the local kids hang out or where there's a territorial aggressive dog. And don't forget to think about the weather – runners suffer sunburn too and if there's any wind it's always easier to set out against the wind and run back with it behind you.

47. Let's get positive

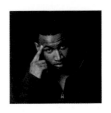

Better sex, sharper mind, longer life – managed right, stress does it all.

Believe it or not, some stress is necessary.
Why? For a start, feeling 'stressy' once or twice a week makes your adrenal glands produce just the right amount of the hormone dehydroepiandrosterone – known as DHEA to its friends.

What DHEA can do for you
DHEA is thought to build collagen and elastin, stimulating a younger appearance. In tests, mice given DHEA lived longer and had more luxuriant coats. It makes your mind sharper too; short-term stress can make your brain work better. And it can even improve your sex life: women with a low libido who were given doses of DHEA got more interested again.

And there's more
If you're feeling down, a little stress can be just what you need to perk you up again. Stress forces you to make decisions and take responsibility. A

Here's an idea for you ...

Relaxation is easier in the dark. To destress instantly, put your palms over your eyes, shut them and imagine you are enveloped in black velvet.

Defining idea ...

'I took a speed reading course and read War and Peace in 20 minutes – it involves Russia.'
WOODY ALLEN

recent study found that short doses of the stress hormone cortisol protect some people against depression just as anti-depressants regulate mood.

One study showed that people with few pressures are up to 50% more likely to die within ten years of quitting work than those facing major responsibility. People under regular pressure tend to take better control and suffer fewer conditions linked to failing finances, poor relationships and employment problems.

Humans are designed to have occasional short, sharp periods of stress: these give us the 'high' that is necessary for psychological good health. If your life is free of stress you may look to get the highs elsewhere and indulge in 'high-risk behaviour': extreme sports, football hooliganism, drugs. Stress keeps us from falling into bad or, frankly, mad habits.

Learn to manage stress, and use it to your advantage. It will motivate, energise and spur you on to a richer and more fulfilling life.

48. Get on yer bike

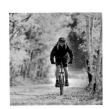

It's difficult to injure yourself cycling because it's such a low-impact form of exercise, plus it's a great way to tone your legs and the nicest way to see the countryside.

Cycling will also strengthen your heart, lower your blood pressure, boost your energy, burn off extra fat and reduce stress. But before you saddle up, do these two things.

Get warmed up
Some cyclists, particularly those of you who hop on your bikes and cycle to work, rarely bother to warm up. If this is you, your main thigh muscle has a high chance of being damaged. Watch out for tight hamstrings and pulled hip too. A heel dig stretch might help as a basic exercise to help all three of these common muscle problems. Simply lift your toes, keep-

Here's an idea for you ...

If cycling gets your wheels turning consider combining it with a holiday. Find a company that'll give you an itinerary suited to your energy level plus accompanying cars to drop off your baggage at the next hotel on the route, then all you'll have to do is pedal and enjoy the view.

Defining idea ...

'Ride lots.'
EDDIE MERCKX

ing your knee straight and your heel on the ground, until you feel a pull in the back and front of the calf and upper thigh.

Get the right bike

- Your choice of bike depends on what you want your bike for. Get some expert advice at a good bike shop and don't be tempted by what looks flashest, prettiest or coolest alone.

- Mountain bikes are rarely suitable for riding in town and that goes for racing bikes too – having your head down when you ride is a sure way of going headlong into a bus!

- Swallow saddles (www.brooksengland.com) are back in vogue, but offer an experience a bit like sitting on a knife. Instead, look for a three-layered saddle of gel/foam/elastic to reduce the pressure on the prostate and pubic bones (www.lookin.it). Aaah, that's more like it!

49. Honey, I'm home!

A spoonful of sugar helps the medicine go down, but a spoonful of honey helps soothe ailments too – especially if it's local.

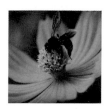

Bees are clever little things. If a bee finds a particularly good source of nectar, it flies the shortest route back to the hive. Bees are also very generous and tell the other bees where to find the nectar by performing a dance routine. You could gain from being generous and clever too, by buying and enjoying some of their delicious produce.

Awareness of the benefits of honey is not new. Honey was one of the most common ingredients in medicines in Ancient Egypt. Honey can help to fight infection because of its antibacterial properties, and it's often used to treat burns and open wounds. Researchers from New Zealand have suggested that honey made from the manuka flower could be used to treat stomach ulcers. Honey is a good cure for hangovers too, since it's high content of sugar helps speed up the processing of alcohol by the liver.

Here's an idea for you ...

If you don't like your honey too upfront, try it mixed with warm water or added to your breakfast cereal.

Defining idea …

'The only reason for being a bee is to
make honey. And the only reason for
making honey is so I can eat it.'
WINNIE THE POOH

So enjoy your honey and consider this.
If you think that you cover a lot of
miles in your job then spare a thought
for the bees, who will have to fly about
55,000 miles to make just one pound
of honey.

Locally-produced honey helps with hayfever too. Just why it works
is still not precisely understood, but popular belief goes something
like this. The pollen local to where you live is often the main trigger
for your hayfever attack. Local honey also contains these irritating
pollens, caught up in the nectar collected by the bees. By giving your
body a regular tiny dose of the pollens that upset you, the honey
helps you build resistance to their effects by teaching it not to react
to them.

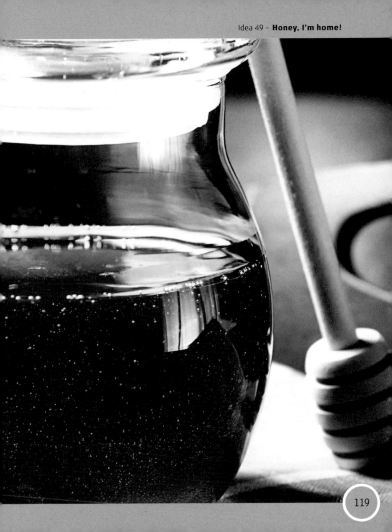

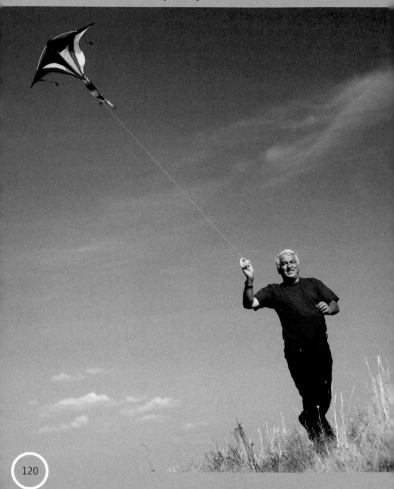

50. Find an hour a day to play

Life really is too short to wallow in the C-list – feeling busy but achieving nothing that matters.

What would you do if you had an hour to yourself every day? The 'desirable' things usually fall into two categories: the stuff we yearn to do because it's fun; and the stuff that's prefixed with 'ought to'. In the first category is lying in bed watching a movie; in the second going for a run or quality time with the kids. We need to find the time for both.

'Life dreams', like writing a novel or learning Russian, fall into the first category. These are 'depth activities' because they add meaning to our lives. And in just an hour a day, you can make a start.

Get the big picture …
Write down everything you're expected to make happen this month, from work projects to socialising, buying birthday presents to decorating. Now go through the list and mark

Here's an idea for you …

On the move and stressed? Running cold water over your wrists for a minute cools you down on a hot day and it works to bring down your stress levels, too.

Defining idea ...

the items you could honestly delegate to someone else. Then decide to hand over 10% of them. By actively thinking about each task and deciding it's something you want to do, you turn it into a choice rather than a chore. Big difference.

Now think about dumping 10% of what you have to do every day. Jot down your 'tasks' for tomorrow. Quickly, without thinking too much, mark them:

A Must do
B Should do
C Could do

Now knock two of the Bs off the list and three of the Cs off and put down in their place an activity that you know would destress you or add depth to your life. Mark it with a whacking great 'A.' Soon, giddy with success, you'll be prioritising yourself all of the time. Well, at least for an hour a day.

51. Be beside the seaside

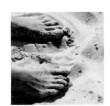

We all feel better at the seaside. But you don't have to be anywhere near the sea to get the benefits.

Donkey rides, buckets and spades, the smell of the ocean. Just thinking about the seaside helps your mind relax. You feel happy because it probably brings back many wonderful childhood memories – unless your overwhelming memory is of being lost and waiting in the beach inspector's office while he tried to summon your parents over the public address system. If you are relaxed, you're likely to be happier and healthier, but there's more to the seaside than this.

For centuries the benefits of sea water have been recognised, with people flocking to the sea to 'take of the water'. But the air is special too. The moisture in sea air 'gets up your nose' and helps to clear it of debris, such as pollen and mucus. If you've ever tried learning to water-ski and taken a dive face first, you'll know precisely how well the sea water can flush out the nasal passages!

Defining idea ...

'The cure for anything is salt water:
sweat, tears or the sea.'
ISAK DINESEN, Danish author

Cleaning the nose and lessening congestion allows the nose to function more effectively. Moreover, trace elements in the sea water are believed to help relieve and prevent the symptoms of nasal allergy – congestion, running and swelling.

No, you don't have to move to the coast to reap the benefits. You can get at least some of the same benefits wherever you live with a seawater micro-spray. These sprays contain – yes, you've guessed it –real seawater. So as you gaze at seaside photographs or TV programmes, spray one up each nostril in turn. Aaah. Isn't that bracing?

And of course, if you can, make a real trip to the seaside. Walk along the beach, listen to the seagulls, enjoy an ice-cream and breathe. Deep breaths. Even a day's break will give your body and mind the most wholesome of holidays.

52. Retreat!

If life, work and the universe in general have become too much, take yourself away from it all and hide (for a while).

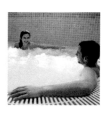

Regeneration and relaxation are incredibly important to health. Yes, there's the doing (exercise, eating right, etc.), but there's just being too. Sometimes we need to slow down if we are to get the balance required for a healthy mind and body – and there's nowhere better to do that than a retreat

Retreats are all about putting your wellbeing first for a while. Since your value to others is radically reduced if you're not 'good within your own skin', don't see this as a purely selfish thing. It's for the benefit of friends and family too.

Try checking out a few of these:

- *www.healthoasisresort.com*
  For those who prefer a beach-front resort, the Health Oasis Resort could be just the ticket.

Here's an idea for you ...

You don't have to go to Thailand to retreat. Find a spa day locally or learn massage at home – look at www. nealsyardremedies.com for oils to practise with.

125

Defining idea ...

'Health is wealth.'
Anonymous

Based in Koh Samui, Thailand, their programmes are designed to promote self-healing in the body and include cleansing, fasting, pampering and colonics (all optional!).

- *www.resortstowellness.com*
  This site lists spas by location and spa type (e.g. lifestyle or cityscape). The focus here is on the individual and they have a very informative section on Executive Health.

- *www.ayurveda.org*
  If five-star luxury is your thing, this isn't the resort for you. Set in the Indian countryside, this retreat offers detox, anti-aging and stress packages using Ayurvedic methods.

- *www.hippocratesinst.org*
  In lush, sunny Florida, this resort offers an impressive range of programmes, including Lifechange, which focuses on education about nutrition and lifestyle.

- *www.aspatolife.com*
  A guide to spas throughout Europe and Barbados. There is an extensive list of treatments, many water-based and all with the emphasis on restoring balance to the body and promoting body-awareness.

- *www.templespa.ie*
  An Irish country house on the site of an ancient monastery, the focus here is on relaxation and wellbeing, with a choice of massages, hot stone therapy and reflexology.

This book is published by Infinite Ideas, creators of the acclaimed **52 Brilliant Ideas** series. If you found this book helpful, here are some other titles in the **Brilliant Little Ideas** series which you may also find interesting.

- **Be incredibly creative:** 52 brilliant little ideas to hone your mind
- **Catwalk looks:** 52 brilliant little ideas to look gorgeous always
- **Drop a dress size:** 52 brilliant little ideas to lose weight and stay slim
- **Enjoy great sleep:** 52 brilliant little ideas for bedtime bliss
- **Get fit:** 52 brilliant little ideas to win at the gym
- **Get rid of your gut:** 52 brilliant little ideas for a sensational six pack
- **Healthy children's lunches:** 52 brilliant little ideas for junk-free meals kids will love
- **Incredible sex:** 52 brilliant little ideas to take you all the way
- **Quit smoking for good:** 52 brilliant little ideas to kick the habit
- **Raising young children:** 52 brilliant little ideas for parenting under 5s
- **Relax:** 52 brilliant little ideas to chill out
- **Shape up your bum:** 52 brilliant little ideas for maximising your gluteus

For more detailed information on these books and others published by Infinite Ideas please visit www.infideas.com.

See reverse for order form.

Qty	Title	RRP
	Be incredibly creative	£5.99
	Catwalk looks	£5.99
	Drop a dress size	£5.99
	Enjoy great sleep	£5.99
	Get fit	£5.99
	Get rid of your gut	£4.99
	Healthy children's lunches	£5.99
	Incredible sex	£5.99
	Quit smoking for good	£4.99
	Raising young children	£5.99
	Relax	£5.99
	Shape up your bum	£5.99
	Add £2.49 postage per delivery address	
	Total	

Name ....

Delivery address ....

....

....

E-mail...............................Tel (in case of problems) ....

By post Fill in all relevant details, cut out or copy this page and send along with a cheque made payable to Infinite Ideas. Send to to: *Brilliant Little Ideas*, Infinite Ideas, 36 St Giles, Oxford OX1 3LD. **Credit card orders over the telephone** Call +44 (0) 1865 514 888. Lines are open 9am to 5pm Monday to Friday.

Please note that no payment will be processed until your order has been dispatched. Goods are dispatched through Royal Mail within 14 working days, when in stock. We never forward personal details on to third parties or bombard you with junk mail. The prices quoted are for UK and RoI residents only. If you are outside these areas please contact us for postage and packing rates. Any questions or comments please contact us on 01865 514 888 or email info@infideas.com.